THE NEW MIDDLE AGES

BONNIE WHEELER, *Series Editor*

The New Middle Ages is a series dedicated to transdisciplinary studies of medieval cultures, with particular emphasis on recuperating women's history and on feminist and gender analyses. This peer-reviewed series includes both scholarly monographs and essay collections.

PUBLISHED BY PALGRAVE:

Women in the Medieval Islamic World: Power, Patronage, and Piety
edited by Gavin R. G. Hambly

The Ethics of Nature in the Middle Ages: On Boccaccio's Poetaphysics
by Gregory B. Stone

Presence and Presentation: Women in the Chinese Literati Tradition
by Sherry J. Mou

The Lost Love Letters of Heloise and Abelard: Perceptions of Dialogue in Twelfth-Century France
by Constant J. Mews

Understanding Scholastic Thought with Foucault
by Philipp W. Rosemann

For Her Good Estate: The Life of Elizabeth de Burgh
by Frances A. Underhill

Constructions of Widowhood and Virginity in the Middle Ages
edited by Cindy L. Carlson and Angela Jane Weisl

Motherhood and Mothering in Anglo-Saxon England
by Mary Dockray-Miller

Listening to Heloise: The Voice of a Twelfth-Century Woman
edited by Bonnie Wheeler

The Postcolonial Middle Ages
edited by Jeffrey Jerome Cohen

Chaucer's Pardoner and Gender Theory: Bodies of Discourse
by Robert S. Sturges

Crossing the Bridge: Comparative Essays on Medieval European and Heian Japanese Women Writers
edited by Barbara Stevenson and Cynthia Ho

Engaging Words: The Culture of Reading in the Later Middle Ages
by Laurel Amtower

Robes and Honor: The Medieval World of Investiture
edited by Stewart Gordon

Representing Rape in Medieval and Early Modern Literature
edited by Elizabeth Robertson and Christine M. Rose

Same Sex Love and Desire Among Women in the Middle Ages
edited by Francesca Canadé Sautman and Pamela Sheingorn

Sight and Embodiment in the Middle Ages: Ocular Desires
by Suzannah Biernoff

Listen, Daughter: The Speculum Virginum and the Formation of Religious Women in the Middle Ages
edited by Constant J. Mews

Science, the Singular, and the Question of Theology
by Richard A. Lee, Jr.

Gender in Debate from the Early Middle Ages to the Renaissance
edited by Thelma S. Fenster and Clare A. Lees

Malory's Morte Darthur: *Remaking Arthurian Tradition*
by Catherine Batt

THE SURGEON IN MEDIEVAL ENGLISH LITERATURE

Jeremy J. Citrome

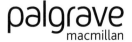

THE SURGEON IN MEDIEVAL ENGLISH LITERATURE
© Jeremy J. Citrome, 2006.

First published in 2006 by
PALGRAVE MACMILLAN™
175 Fifth Avenue, New York, N.Y. 10010 and
Houndmills, Basingstoke, Hampshire, England RG21 6XS
Companies and representatives throughout the world.

PALGRAVE MACMILLAN is the global academic imprint of the Palgrave Macmillan division of St. Martin's Press, LLC and of Palgrave Macmillan Ltd. Macmillan® is a registered trademark in the United States, United Kingdom and other countries. Palgrave is a registered trademark in the European Union and other countries.

ISBN-13: 978–1–4039–6846–3
ISBN-10: 1–4039–6846–2

Library of Congress Cataloging-in-Publication Data

Citrome, Jeremy J.
    The surgeon in medieval English literature / Jeremy J. Citrome.
        p. cm.—(The new Middle Ages)
    Includes bibliographical references and index.
    ISBN 1–4039–6846–2 (alk. paper)
    1. Christian poetry, English (Middle)—History and criticism.
    2. Surgery in literature. 3. Christianity in literature. 4. Literature and
    medicine—England—History—To 1500. 5. English literature—Middle
    English, 1100–1500—History and criticism. I. Title. II. New Middle Ages
    (Palgrave Macmillan (Firm))

PR365.C58 2006
821′.1093561—dc22   2005057635

A catalogue record for this book is available from the British Library.

Design by Newgen Imaging Systems (P) Ltd., Chennai, India.

First edition: September 2006
10 9 8 7 6 5 4 3 2 1

Printed in the United States of America.

For my parents

CONTENTS

ACKNOWLEDGMENTS

This project began life as a doctoral thesis and has undergone several changes along the road to publication. As with any long journey, completion has depended not only on the passion and determination of the traveller, but also on the generosity and patience of the various guides he has met along the way. Indeed, several such guides have helped me to my destination, and I would like to thank each of them: Catherine Batt, for her keen insights and obervations during the doctoral stage of this project and beyond; George R. Keiser, for generously sharing his astounding knowledge of Middle English medical writings; Ann Hutchison, for helping me to understand the wonderful world of later medieval spirituality; Bonnie Wheeler, for her interest in this project from its very first incarnation; and Carole Rawcliffe, for her thoughtful encouragement in the early days and absolutely crucial suggestions in the final ones. I would also like to thank the Pontifical Institute of Mediaeval Studies, whose peerless resources and generous funding allowed me to complete the research for the third chapter of this book. While I cannot thank each conference organizer and co-panelist who has offered invaluable advice over the years, I do want to acknowledge Gerard NeCastro and Bryon Grigsby, whose tireless planning and promoting of Medica events at Kalamazoo have provided myself and others interested in medieval medicine with a forum in which to discuss and improve our work. This book also would not have been possible without the generous permissions of *The Chaucer Review* and *Exemplaria* to print revised versions of, respectively, chapters 1 and 4, which first appeared as articles in those venerable journals. Lastly, I would like to thank, for their endless and indispensable support, my friends Kofi Campbell, Tom Vernon, Danny Landsdell, Carol Weller, and, most importantly of all, my parents, Dr. George and Elaine Citrome.

INTRODUCTION: SURGERY AND
THE WOUNDS OF SIN

> Do we use these as empirically as our predecessors did their leeches and their
> bleedings?. . .Are we, in the light of others who come after us, going to be
> accused of being users of stupid, bizarre or crude methods? Will they think
> us no better than quacks?. . .Will they read our shock therapy methods with
> horror and say, "Why, they should have used baseball bats—it would have
> been just as productive of results"?
>
> Pressman, Last Resort[1]

The above words, spoken in 1941 by the noted psychiatrist
C. Burlinghame in an after-dinner speech to colleagues, illustrate the
folly of regarding the customs of the past from too high a pedestal.
Burlinghame, a pioneer of psychosurgical procedures ranging from shock
treatment to lobotomy, invokes as part of his rhetorical strategy medicine
that is recognizably "medieval," and that modern society tends to either
greet with laughter or dismiss contemptuously. Yet Burlinghame's artless
pillory of medieval surgery betrays an overt anxiety over his own healing
methods. Indeed, the mutilation of the frontal lobe to curtail antisocial
behavior is now regarded as a relic of a particularly inhumane period
of psychiatric medicine. Although Burlinghame employs the perceived
antiquity—indeed, the *alterity*—of medieval surgical methods to make his
own practices seem innovative by comparison, there is, in fact, continuity
at work here. The violence of Burlinghame's methods are designed to rein-
tegrate the patient into the law-abiding community, just as the "leeches,"
"bleedings," and other forceful excisions that constituted medieval surgery
were meant to restore the patient not just physically but also morally and
spiritually. To the profoundly penitential culture of later medieval England,
sin and sickness were inextricably linked; and surgery, even as it progressed
in its ability to cure physical affliction, became even more important as a
metaphor for the pursuit of spiritual health. This book therefore attempts
to tell two stories. The first is that of the surgeon's rapid emergence as a figure
of literary significance in the fourteenth century; the second is his simultaneous

transformation into both religious metaphor and psychological agent by an institution of unprecedented cultural influence. To tell these two stories is not a work of medical history, nor an exercise in literary criticism, but an examination of the social power of metaphor as it affected English society in the later Middle Ages. In this introduction, I will demonstrate the central fact that made the surgeon so convenient a metaphor for the urgent struggle between damnation and salvation that resided at the heart of medieval Christian identity: surgery, because it both healed and hurt, could uniquely signify the profound ambivalence, the tension between merciful and punitive registers, that constituted humanity's relationship with the divine in the English Middle Ages.

Surgery had long been marginalized in classical and scholastic definitions of medicine as the last possible resort in a threefold hierarchy of healing strategies. According to the eleventh-century Arabic authority Avicenna, whose great work *The Canon of Medicine* was translated into Latin by Gerard of Cremona in Toledo in the twelfth century and parts of which became indispensable to the university medical syllabus, the "subject of treatment comprises three headlines: that of regimen and diet, that of the use of medicines, and that of manual operative interference."[2] Despite its status as the ultimate method, which was to be employed only once diet and drugs had failed, surgery shared in the same theoretical framework as did the rest of medical treatment: that of the four humors. This ancient physiological theory was first made famous by Hippocrates and his followers, elaborated by Galen in the second century, and then transmitted to the Latin West through scholastic translations of Arabic intermediaries. It held that the universe was composed of four distinct elements—fire, air, water, and earth—which our bodies convert through digestion into four biological liquids, or humors: melancholy, phlegm, blood, and choler. Each of us possesses an innate humoral combination, or *complexion*, that helps determine our entire range of physical and psychological attributes. However, due to human imperfection these humors are unstable and can become dangerously unbalanced. Superfluous humors that we cannot excrete through natural means must be adjusted medically if we are to remain healthy. Medical treatments revolve around either the regulation of these humors through diet and drugs or their manual purgation through a variety of invasive methods, which Avicenna lists as "blood-letting, wet-cupping, purgation, enemas, diaphoresis, use of leeches, etc."[3] For the administering physician, such violent treatments involving the cutting and scarring of the flesh or the either partial or whole amputation of a limb are difficult as these methods are "not appreciated as such by the patient because of the pain and suffering they cause him until the symptom has been removed."[4] Yet until the thirteenth century, this anxiety that attended surgical treatment was absorbed into, and diluted by, the harmoniously unified nature of the three parts of medicine, each of which was included in the trained physician's arsenal. With the Fourth Lateran Council of 1215, however, medicine underwent a fragmentation that results not only in the emergence of the professional surgeon as an autonomous figure but also in his widely influential transformation into spiritual metaphor.

The Fourth Lateran Council has assumed special importance for historians of both medical and devotional history. At this council, Pope Innocent III put into effect a variety of reforms that were meant to prohibit the clergy from secular activity. Surgery was among these pursuits Innocent identified as dissonant with the clerical vocation. Because of this ruling, surgery became separated discursively, though not always practically, from the prescription of drugs and dietary regulation.[5] Within the same edict, however, other prohibitions occur that are only seemingly unrelated. Apart from the reasons that the cleric in major orders should not practice surgery—mainly its potential for secular profit, incompatible with Catholic Church teachings—he also should not preside in any way over torture, ordeals, or, indeed, any activity that leads to the shedding of blood.[6] Without a doubt, however, the most important development to occur at this council is the consolidation of confession as a mandatory requirement for all Christians.[7] Not to confess at least once a year would now result in excommunication, effectively bringing all parishioners under the spiritual authority of the Church. With the advent of mandatory auricular confession, the thirteenth century saw the emergence of a new form of selfhood. Although private confession had existed throughout the Middle Ages, and was explicated in manuals of Celtic origin since the sixth century, it had hitherto been performed only sporadically and was often delayed until the moment of death. As Mary Braswell has documented, the conflict that arose in early-thirteenth-century England between Innocent and King John plunged the country into a state of spiritual impoverishment. In England under interdict, Mass, along with other points of Christian observance, was largely forgotten.[8] Bishops returning from the Fourth Lateran Council became aware of the immensity of the project before them, namely, the reeducation of priests and parishioners in the fundamentals of Christian observance.[9] The result was the massive proliferation of vernacular manuals of confession for priests and laypeople alike, and with them a new language of penance that would have the effect of distinguishing the speaking subject from the collective, communal identity. Because of the unique situation in England, parishioners were required to confess their sins not once but three times a year.[10] This, combined with the rapid dissemination of vernacular penitential literature, ensured that parishioners there were more thoroughly exposed to the language of post-Lateran penance than were those elsewhere in Western Christendom. As Jerry Root has demonstrated, it was through such sheer repetition that confession was able "to codify and make available a convenient grid, a limited discursive space in which medieval penitents may present themselves."[11] The profoundly reiterative nature of confession after the Fourth Lateran Council created a performative context in which parishioners could articulate their most transgressive and individuating desires frequently, precisely, and over an extended period of time. However, such liberating individuation was not an end in itself but a passing moment in the greater project in which penitent and confessor worked together to "transform the space of the world into the space of grace."[12] Indeed, pastoral writers often encouraged their audience to confess more frequently than the annual absolution Innocent demanded of parishioners at Lent. John Myrk, the late-fourteenth-century priest and sermonizer, instructs the reader of his *Festial* to be "schryuen of his synnys" not only "from lenton to lenton, but as sone as he feleþe þat he hath synnet," urging him to "mekly take þe dome of his schryft-fadyr" just as a "knyght scheweth þe wondys þat he haþe yn bataylle."[13] Taken together, these references to wounds, penance, and parental authority assume a rhetorical power that pastoral writers most frequently accessed through a single, highly charged metaphor—the surgeon- confessor.

While to an extent Innocent's ban on the higher orders shedding blood merely consolidated surgery's debased position as the least prestigious of available treatments, it also helped to establish it as an autonomous profession by effectively designating its bloody work to the ranks of the lay population. Innocent's demand at this same council that physicians summon priests to the bedsides of the terminally ill before operating themselves further established, according to Joseph Ziegler, "strict boundaries between the physicians of the body and those of the soul."[14] Because, as Innocent asserts, "sickness of the body may sometimes be the result of sin," patients must first consult "physicians of the soul so that after their spiritual health has been seen to they may respond better to medicine for their bodies; for when the cause ceases so does the effect."[15] Yet remarkably, despite the undeniable negativity of this canon toward earthly medicine, the previous canon, which relates to confession, compares this new *sine qua non* of salvation to the most mundane and earthly operation imaginable: the surgical treatment of a wound. As Innocent declares,

> The priest shall be discerning and prudent, so that like a skilled doctor he may pour wine over the wounds of the injured one. Let him carefully enquire about the circumstances of both the sinner and the sin, so that he may prudently discern what sort of advice he ought to give and what remedy to apply, using various means to heal the sick person.[16]

Although Innocent may have had in mind the Good Samaritan of the New Testament, the medical technique that he describes belongs explicitly to this third, and most dangerous, branch of medicine: the simple application of wine, was the dominant mode of wound treatment in the thirteenth century. Indeed, the fourteenth-century French surgical practitioner and author Guy de Chauliac dismissively characterizes his predecessors as those who "drieden indifferently alle woundes wiþ wyne alone."[17] Surgery emerges from this dual appropriation of the literal and the metaphorical as an ambivalent art, at once both consonant and dissonant with ecclesiastical notions of spiritual health. Metaphors of surgery become the key rhetorical device through which subsequent pastoral writers explain spiritual health in this reinforced confessional context, and the surgeon, their foremost model for the perfect confessor. Later examples involve far more complex treatments than that which Innocent describes, a development facilitated by the simultaneous explosion in the fourteenth century of Middle English manuals of confession and surgery. Occasionally these parallel discourses converged materially, for example, in the form of priests who translated Latin works of surgery for guild-oriented surgeons too poor to afford or commission their own versions of prominent textbooks, some of whom even practiced themselves.[18] Indeed, Irma Taavitsainen and Päivi Pahta have recently demonstrated the possible existence of a scriptorium in either London or the East Midlands that specialized in both devotional and surgical manuscripts.[19] Given these simultaneous developments, it is no wonder that surgery thrives as spiritual metaphor in the centuries following the Fourth Lateran Council.

The fact that the wounded body of this passage so obviously belongs to the realm of metaphor should not lead us to ignore the existence of an integral connection, on a literal level, between the medieval concepts of sin and sickness. To do so would be to ignore the causal relationship thought to exist between the two, and that helped to render the medieval surgeon so remarkable a figure of ambivalence. To a medieval patient, illness and its subsequent treatment must have seemed a microcosm of Original Sin and *its* treatment through the intervention of Christ. At the simplest level, successful surgery depended on the presence of divine grace, which St. Augustine of Hippo famously demonstrated in his harrowing account of the healing of the counsellor Innocentius in *The City of God*. According to the towering theologian, the pious Innocentius suffered from ulcers of the anus that his skilled surgeons painfully healed, all except for one located so deep in the rectum that it would have required a potentially fatal operation had God not responded with a miraculous cure to the prayers of Augustine and his company.[20] On the more complicated level of physiology, however, the external afflictions surgery so painfully corrected were often considered the direct result of immoral behavior. An ancient Greek tradition related to that of the humors, one emerging with the Stoics and expanded by the famed Arabic physician Rhazes, identified three bodily spirits, or functions of the soul, that move the human organism: the natural spirit, the crudest of the three, generates in the liver and governs growth, nutrition, and reproduction; the vital spirit, which the heart creates by heating the natural spirits in the blood, animates the organism with life; and the animal spirit, located in the brain and composed of vital spirits combined with air breathed in through the nostrils, provides intellect, sensation, and voluntary motion.[21] Although the animal spirit seems the most important, it is in fact the second of these three quasi-ethereal substances, the vital spirit, that is most essential to overall health, for without the invigorating heat it produces all bodily powers would fail. The various excesses of passion Christian theologians would have recognized as sin—for example, wrath or despair—can affect the body directly by causing this vital heat to either rush from the heart to the extremities, leading to visible afflictions, or withdraw to the heart, causing paralysis. To ensure that such heat dispersed in good proportion, the physician had to make certain that the biological fluids that comprise the body, the four humors, held their own corresponding balance.[22] As we shall see, one way this balance was maintained was through the regulation of such external factors as diet, sleep, and sexual behavior.

Indeed, theologians had long favored an explanation of the Fall that took into account the same humoral pathology at work in everyday afflictions. The twelfth-century abbess Hildegard of Bingen provides an especially thorough discussion of this relationship between postlapsarian imperfection and humoral imbalance. According to Hildegard, "if the human had remained in Paradise he would not have in his body those *flegmata* leading to many evils but, rather, his flesh would be undamaged," but, because of Original Sin, "their flesh is ulcerous and perforated."[23] This degradation of the humors initiated in the Fall is the primary cause of all subsequent illness. The thirteenth-century Franciscan Friar Roger Bacon, for example, developed an entire medical system based on the premise of this original corruption. According to Bacon, Original Sin created within us an innate physical vulnerability that shortens the natural duration of human life:

> For sins weaken the powers of the soul, so that it is incompetent for the natural control of the body; and therefore the powers of the body are weakened and life is shortened. This weakening passes from father to son, and so on. Therefore owing to these two natural causes the longevity of man of necessity has not retained its natural course from the beginning; but for these two reasons the longevity of man has been shortened contrary to nature.[24]

We are caught in a vicious circle: unbalanced in our humors, we are too weak to resist sin, and our continued transgressions remove us ever further from our prelapsarian selves. Although Bacon recommends the ingestion of simple medicines, it is only through salvation that we can regain that internal cohesion, the "equality of elements" that now can only "exist in our bodies after the resurrection."[25] In a very real sense, then, wounds and other signs of illness are not merely metaphors for spiritual corruption, but they are the material substance of sin manifest upon the flesh.

The surgeon cured such blemishes through a variety of violent methods, including burning, cutting, and the application of corrosive chemicals. He therefore accrued strong penitential resonances, not only as metaphor for the spiritual ministrations of the clergy but also in his own right. Indeed, the Middle English version of the *Chirurgia* of the twelfth-century Italian surgeon Roger of Parma conflates physical and spiritual healing by insisting that it is "Ihu crist that is the principal leche of mennys bodyes and also of ther soules."[26] In a similar vein, the famed fourteenth-century Newark surgeon John Arderne, in the Middle English version of his *Practica*, compares the obedience the patient owes the surgeon to that which humanity owes Christ:

> [I]f paciente3 pleyne þat ther medicine3 ben bitter or scharpe or siche othir than schalt the leche sey to the pacyent þat it is redde in the last seson of matyne of the natiuite of our lorde that cryst come in to this worlde for the helpe of mane3 kynd to the maner of a good leche and wise and when he comeþ to the seke man he scheweþ hym medicyne3 some light and some harde and he seythe to the sekeman if thou wilt be made hole þise and þise schalt thou take. . .[27]

John Arderne overtly connects the painful ministrations of the surgeon to the corrections of the Son, our first spiritual "leche," whose abstemious model of living requires as much patience, discipline, and discretion as does undergoing the most grueling surgical operation. The rise of surgery as an autonomous profession introduces into the rhetoric of spiritual health an unmistakably punitive component, in keeping with the overarching motif that damnation—with its attendant pains of hell—is the ultimate punishment for failing to confess one's sins. Just as surgery could stand for the eternal bodily wholeness that is the reward of salvation, it could also stand for its opposite: the eternal fragmentation that characterizes the bodies of the damned in the Middle English penitential tradition. According to one widely available Northumbrian treatise, *The Pricke of Conscience*, the saved are eternally "semely and bright" in the afterlife, while the damned "sal alle unsemely be," and even "foul, and ugly, opon to se."[28] Surgery, because it can replicate either of these eschatological states, possesses a remarkable plasticity as metaphor, and it can uniquely convey, by way of earthly example, the sometimes uneasy relationship between mercy and punishment that resides in the rhetoric of confession. This relationship derives not only from the rhetoric of confession but also from its history. As John Baldwin has demonstrated, the bloodless confessional practices made mandatory in the Fourth Lateran Council do not represent a sharp departure from previous, more violent methods of eliciting obedience, but rather an evolution of those same principles of making Church power manifest. The ecclesiastical ordeal, writes Baldwin, "continued to embody the exercise of God's power up to the eve of the Council," where confession was confirmed at the same time as the ordeal was condemned.[29] The most common forms of ordeal involved gripping the hot iron, immersing the hand in boiling water, and walking across hot plowshares. Injury amounts to evidence of concealed guilt on the part of the accused. The following excerpt from a thirteenth-century breviary illustrates this connection between the ordeal and the sacrament of confession that replaced it:

> O clement and most holy Ruler, give aid if he shall plunge his hand into the boiling water, being innocent, and, as Thou didst liberate the three youths from the fiery furnace and didst free Susanna from the false charge, so, O Lord, bring forth his hand safe and unharmed from this water. But if he be guilty and presume to plunge in his hand, the devil hardening his heart, let Thy holy justice deign to declare it, that Thy virtue may be manifest in his body and his soul be saved by penitence and confession. And if the guilty man shall try to hide his sins by the use of herbs or any magic, let Thy right hand deign to bring it to no account. Through Thy only begotten Son, our Lord Jesus Christ, who dwelleth with Thee.[30]

In both the ordeal and auricular confession, the objective is to uncover sins that the subject is attempting to hide, thus purifying the transgressor. Where the former involves actual, physical violence, the latter employs the discursive representation thereof. Indeed, penitential literature often emphasizes the painful consequences of damnation in ways reminiscent of both torture and surgical treatment. For example, the fifteenth-century sermon collection *Jacob's Well* illustrates the importance of confession through the tale of Ode, whose soul after death is subjected to an "yren leep all glowynge as fyir" until it "roryd for peyne."[31] The author then warns us, with uncontained exuberance, that if we "dyest wyth-oute repentauns," we, too, "schalt be bathyd, as Ode was, in brennyng pych & oyle!"[32] Similarly, the confessional manual contained within the *Cursor mundi* compares damnation to "a glouande irin" inserted "þoru þi limis alle."[33] This last example alludes to the torture device of the hot iron, another key tool in the ecclesiastical ordeal. The presence of so specific an ethos of torture in confessional manuals is not surprising, given the close historical relationship between the ordeal and private confession. By comparing themselves to surgeons, who in England were always secular figures, confessors could retain a suggestion of the ordeal's coercive violence, while avoiding associations, condemned in the Fourth Lateran Council, between clergy and literal bloodshed. After all, the "glowande irin" of the *Cursor mundi* is more than a little reminiscent of the surgical cautery, which William of Touke describes as "an yron glowynge hote."[34] The *Fasciculus Morum* makes this association between surgical pain and sin explicit when it recommends, as a cure for lechery, "the cautery of chastity."[35] Such painful yet healing associations serve to render both surgeon and confessor figures of remarkable ambivalence. The surgeon promises health, but this promise is fulfilled at the cost of suffering great pain. The confessor enables the achievement of salvation but only through the discomfort of painful and humiliating admissions. That this latter sacrifice is so frequently figured as surgical pain suggests that confession seeks to associate itself not only with the surgeon's healing capacity but also with the painful nature of his craft. The confessor displaces his own punitive force onto the figure of the surgeon, thereby mitigating the tensions that arise from his uneasy conflation of merciful and punitive registers. Nowhere is this ambivalence more evident than in the most common of all surgical metaphors: the wounds of sin.

The surgical metaphor of sin as a wound can be broken down into three components. First, an abundance of humoral matter forms within the body and is expelled to the surface of the flesh, where the humors collect and gradually corrupt. Second, a wound forms at this location, requiring a diagnostic examination by the surgeon to determine its type and severity. Third, the wound must be treated, either by incision, burning iron, or the application of corrosive chemicals, or a drawing salve. In confessional rhetoric, the corresponding actions generally involve the buildup of sinful thoughts and behavior, the confessor's subsequent inquisition of the confessant, and finally the painful admission of sins leading ultimately to the absolution that heals the sinner. The careful assembly in many confessional manuals of extant surgical knowledge bespeaks an awareness among priests and parishioners alike of, at the very least, the rudiments of practical medical treatment. The ubiquity of surgery in later medieval society, along with the concurrent translations of confessional and surgical treatises into Middle English, meant that the intersections between spiritual and physical discourses were newly strengthened, crystallizing in the metaphor of the surgeon-confessor.

The first component of this metaphor, the formation of the wound, turns on the concept of the humors and their corruption. One or other of these biological fluids collects at a certain location on the body, stagnates, and then decays, causing a wound to form. Humors are the primary substance of the body, both forming the limbs and providing their nourishment, and their corruption is the primary cause of all physical illness. A Middle English translation of Galen's *De ingenio sanitatis*, the theoretical foundation for its predominantly surgical manuscript,[36] emphasizes the absolute centrality of humoral theory to all diagnosis and treatment of wounds:

> If a wounde be made in any membres of any maner mater we understonde wele þat it shuld noȝt be bot of yuel humors. ffor why: custome of nature is for to make þingȝ in passions. þat is to sey, it mundifieþ þe body and putteþ out wiþout þe skynne.[37]

The development of a wound therefore signals a preceding, internal corruption. As John Gaddesden, the thirteenth-century English physician and author of the influential compendium *Rosa Anglica* puts it, "Since a humour is peccant in every sickness in the world, if the matter be harmful, the member is injured."[38] This specter of internal corruption contributes to the power of the wound to signify moral turpitude. Indeed, even on a literal level the humoral character of wounds does not divest the patient of responsibility for his or her compromised state. Such corruption is often said to arise from intemperate use of the body, which shifts its contents and causes dangerous imbalances to occur. Following an ancient tradition, medieval practitioners prescribed strict regulation of the body through the proper governing of the six "nonnaturals," roughly equivalent to what we might today call "lifestyle." The fifteenth-century Italian surgeon Berengario da Carpi lists these variables as air, motion and rest, food and drink, sleep and waking, digestion and constipation, and emotions. If the individual exercises moderation in these, he "will preserve his natural condition and strengthen his health until his natural death," but if "he behaves otherwise than he should in these matters he perishes and if he is already ill his illness is worsened and increased."[39] Indeed, medical practitioners frequently instructed their patients to avoid a range of activities identical to the sins that they would customarily have confessed to their parish priests. Da Carpi himself commands post-operative patients to avoid lechery, because coitus "resolves or diminishes the innate heat and destroys bodily power if it is superfluous,"[40] while Gaddesden describes those requiring phlebotomy as gluttonous, "the people that fill themselves excessively and are drunken, who cannot but have crude humors."[41] So dangerous is lecherous behavior to the maintenance of the body that, according to the plague tract of John of Burgundy, one should "fle soueraignly huntyng of lechery fore that bothe openes the pores and destroies the kinde naturel and also enfebles þe spirituell membres and also the lyvely spirites in a man."[42] The wound therefore contains an inescapably moral dimension; immoderation gives way to internal imbalances, which then create disturbances across the surface of the body. Penitential writers understood the role of humors in the commission of sin; the anonymous author of the *Speculum Sacerdotale*, for example, explains the importance of fasting as the method by which "we schuld refreyne these fowre humours fro synnynge."[43] The "wounds of sin" are therefore at once both metaphorical and literal, an interdependence of mind and flesh that facilitates the incorporation of the surgeon into the rhetoric of confession.

Indeed, surgeons often attend to the souls of their patients at the same time as they do their bodies. Da Carpi, in obedience to Innocent's privileging of spiritual over physical medicine, prioritizes confession as the ultimate cure:

> The patient should be advised at the first visit of the physician that he should confess his sins to God. . .since the illness is often produced by reason of those sins before the doctor of souls is called because thus excommunication is avoided. In this way patients are healed better and more quickly from many causes of illness.[44]

One cannot help but notice the tension in the margins of this passage. While da Carpi appears to endorse Innocent's influential canon concerning the primacy of confession, the foremost operation of spiritual healing, over earthly medicine, he also suggests that fear of punishment, specifically excommunication, motivates such obedience. Surgeons frequently discussed not only the formative effects of sin on the development of illness but also the quality of divine retribution that inheres in disease and its treatment. The surgeon, like the priest, becomes a disciplinary agent of God. Roger of Parma, for example, asserts that the underlying cause of many illnesses is that God "maketh schrewes syke to withdraw hem from her shrewdness and to make hem thynk on hym in her syknes that ne wole not thynke on hym."[45] In the same manuscript, John of Burgundy's plague tract warns that the cause of pestilence is often "vengeaunce taking for syn," and the cure, confession: "for euery man in what degre other what estate that he be putte a wey syn thorgh verry sorowe and contricion asking of god mekely and also foryeuenesse with shrift of mouth, satisfaccion werking, and eke penaunce doing fore his syn."[46] The buildup of corrupt humors at the surface of the flesh correlates roughly to the amount of sinful behavior that the patient engages in: the greater the immoderation and consequent movement of the humors, the greater the quantity of corrupt matter to be expelled from the wound. As Lanfranco states, the intention of the surgeon is to eradicate, through the knife, burning iron, or corrosive chemical, the "manye superfluytees þat beþ nouȝt semelich to mannys body."[47] Surgery therefore functions as a painful check to libidinal excess, cutting away at the physical manifestations of sin just as the priest, according to the confessional manual *Of Shrifte and Penance*, must excise spiritual corruption to make "a mannus soule evene."[48] The wounds of sin, then, are the physical inscription of sin upon the body, an earthly reminder of the fragmenting punishments that await the bodies of the damned—including the excommunicated—in the afterlife.

The second component of the "wounds of sin" metaphor, diagnosis, facilitates this displacement of ecclesiastical power onto the figure of the surgeon by replicating confession's verbal methodology. Once a wound appears, it falls to the surgeon to plan an appropriate course of action. Wounds were of many varieties. They could be either simple or compound—that is, superficial or breaching the sinews—and required different treatments depending upon their depth, degree of corruption, and location on the body. These factors determine whether a surgeon should employ incision or the less invasive methods of potential or actual cautery. The difference between the potential and actual cautery is of chemical- and fire-induced heat, or, in the words of the Middle English Galen, "brynnyng medicine or brynnyng of fire."[49] Because an error in surgery is seldom repairable, the failure to determine treatment in this fashion is the sign of a bad or untrained practitioner. Surgeons undertake this essential diagnosis of a wound in two ways: through visual examination of the afflicted area, and by the verbal inquisition of the patient. The Middle English Galen recommends both these exploratory avenues before deciding on a treatment, instructing the surgeon to both "serch and inquire sekenes."[50] Saliceto, as well, conflates verbal with tactile diagnosis, instructing the surgeon to proceed "be wey of inquisicion or serchinge."[51] As Edward Peter has demonstrated, ecclesiastical inquisitions often employed the threat of physical torture, in which "the accused might be shown the instruments of torture in order to obtain a confession quickly, particularly from the apprehensive or faint-hearted."[52] In this sense, medieval surgery shares with ecclesiastical inquisition the effect of, as Elaine Scarry has stated of modern torture, "dramatizing the connection between two dreaded forms of exposure, open wounds and confession."[53] Michel Foucault too has noted in *The History of Sexuality* that torture "has accompanied confession like a shadow, and supported it when it could go no further." The medieval surgeon was aware of the power of his own instruments to invoke the fear of bodily pain. We find in John Arderne's *Practica* an acknowledgment of this same fearful relationship between verbal inquisition and the display of painful instruments:

> When þe leche, forsoþe, haþ talked þus to þe pacient, as it is seid, and þe
> pacient aske and persew for to be cured of hym, aske þan first þe siȝt of
> þe sekenes; Whiche y-sene, be þe leche war þat he put noȝt his fynger in þe
> lure of þe pacient, ne shewe no pryue instrumenteȝ wher-of þe pacient myȝt
> wonder or be aferd.[54]

The repeated exposure of the patient to penitential rhetoric might well
have caused him to equate the pain signified by these "instrumenteȝ,"
and the interrogation that accompanies them, with the power of the
confessor to bestow or deny absolution. The priest, in adopting the figure
of the surgeon, assumes not only the surgeon's role as healer but also his
associations with pain, discipline, and punishment.

The visual component of diagnosis, like its verbal counterpart, signifies the
confessor's task of eliciting a full and open confession from the parishioner.
According to the anonymous author of the fourteenth-century *The Book of
Vices and Virtues*, a Middle English rendering of the Anglo-Norman *Somme le
roi* written by Friar Laurent in the previous century, the confessor must "see
openliche þe herte and þe vnderstondyng of hym or of hire þat schryueþ
hym," just as "þe leche ne may not hele a wounde but he see openliche al þe
wounde."[55] The widespread use of the surgical tent is central to this comparison. The tent has two functions: opening the wound so that it may be clearly
viewed to the bottom, and holding it in this position so that knife or cautery
can be inserted to maximum depth. Apart from its practical uses, the tent
operates on a theoretical level. The principle of *secondary intention*, despite
having endured a period of debate in the thirteenth century, remained the
dominant theory of wound treatment throughout the Middle Ages. This
theory holds that the wound must heal from the bottom up, in order for
corrupt humors to evacuate the wound for the duration of the healing process.
Roger of Parma, for example, demands that the surgeon ensure "thy tent
be grete aboue that the wound be hole open," for if wounds retain any
corruption, they may be "worsse than they were in the first begynnyng."[56]
The confessional manual contained within the *Cursor mundi* makes use of this
surgical commonplace to signify the importance of frequent and full confession and the damnation that results from the incomplete articulation of sins:

> hit faris of shrift as dos of wound
> þat lange vnsoȝt is to þe grounde
> a tent þe wers to hit wil reche
> quen hit rotis for defaute of leche
> in muche bale hit mai be wroȝt

bot hit wiþ saluing sone be soȝt
hit stinkis rynnis & rotis ay.
wiþ-outen wa wil noȝt a-way.
(ll. 26636–43)

We can thus make a number of comparisons: the discontinuity of the body to the impurity of the soul, the surgeon's deep probing of the wound to the confessor's probing of the conscience, and death through insufficient treatment to damnation by incomplete confession. By associating the urgency of full confession with that of effective surgical treatment, confessors could communicate in terrifyingly visceral fashion the consequences of defying the terms of Innocent's expanded requirements for auricular confession: the excruciating pains of damnation.

The third and final component of the surgical metaphor is the treatment itself, which follows diagnosis and involves some form of painful ministration. In examining a particularly inclusive example of this metaphor from *Jacob's Well*, we have a sense of the ambivalence of this crucial, final stage of both surgery and confession:

[N]ow schal I telle ȝou how ȝe schal caste out þe hard wose of ȝoure synne, þat is þe harde obstynacye of ȝoure synne, wyth a scauel of confessioun. for þat scauel of clene schryfte muste nedys folwe sorwe of herte, ȝyf þou mowe haue a preest, & ellys þou art out of þe weye of saluacyoun. for, þowȝ deed flesch be kut out of a wounde, wyth a scharp corryzie, þi wounde, þowȝ, nedyth to be pourgyd, wyth a drawyng salue; ellys it wolde rotyn and festryn aȝen. Ryȝt so, þowȝ þi dedly synne be kut out, wyth sorwe of herte, fro þe pyt of þi conscyens, ȝit þi conscyens nedyth to be pourgyd, wyth a drawyng salue of clene schryfte, & ellys þe wounde of dedly synne rotyth & festryth aȝen in þi soule.[57]

The author employs an accurate description of medieval wound treatment to illustrate the difference between mere disclosure, an external act, and true repentance, an internal state. The painful application of "corryzie," the potential cautery, stands for the contrition that removes the corrupt "deed flesch" of sin from the heart. Finally, the placing of a "drawyng salue" on the wound signals the conclusion of the treatment, metaphorically the full confession that finally "heals" the sinner. According to John Arderne, such salves cleanse the corruption from wounds by "drawyng fro partieȝ bineþ to aboue," a detail in keeping with the emphasis in this passage on the transformation, through confession, of corrupt desires into the salutary matter of absolution.[58] The sinner is now purged of the corrupting matter of sin and may be assured of the pleasures of salvation. Yet it is clear that confession, like surgery, was a painful operation that required the patience and fortitude of its subjects, and the surgeon, because he embodied both kinds of healing, was often constructed as an uncompromising and unflinching torturer. John Trevisa, for example, insists in his translation of the thirteenth-century encyclopedia *De Propietatibus Rerum* that the ideal surgeon does not stop "keruynge oþir brennynge for wepinge of þe pacient."[59] It is hardly surprising that pastoral writers employed the surgeon in this fashion, given the unavoidably harrowing experience of undergoing practical medical treatment in this period. According to Lanfranco, the surgeon's duty mainly comprises "kuttynge or openynge" corrupt matter, and "doynge awey þat is to myche."[60] Amputation was a common penitential motif even outside of references to surgery, and it was used to signify the process of abandoning those behaviors that exclude us from grace. The fifteenth-century sermon collection *Speculum Sacerdotale*, for example, recommends that we "cutteþ a-way þese vices," including "oure hertis þat we thynke non evel" and "oure feet fro evel wayes."[61] The fourteenth-century preacher's handbook *Fasciculus Morum* assimilates the surgeon into this motif, urging "the surgical removal of evil companionship and the occasion of sin."[62] Such passages correspond well to Trevisa's description of the uncompromising surgeon, demonstrating the interdependence of the experiential and the metaphorical in both the social construction of the surgeon and his appropriation for didactic purposes in writings on confession.

In their desire to associate confession with the bitter yet healing pains of surgery, religious writers tended to understate the range of treatments that figured prominently in the regimen. Medieval surgeons were by no means limited to cutting and burning. Many surgeons employed medicinal baths in order to relieve pain and encourage the patient's body to sweat out its corruption, and nearly all acted as their own apothecaries in order to fashion soothing ointments for dermatological conditions.[63] Indeed, although patient testimonials are rare in this period, the surgical literature does suggest a rather more merciful figure than Trevisa's stern abstraction, and the continued insistence outside of surgical discourses on the harsh, discomfiting surgeon can be regarded as largely a fictive yet strategic construction. While they were not exactly dispensing lollipops to brave patients, much of the evidence does support a picture of medieval practitioners as generally compassionate, as much as this is possible within the confines of this paradigmatically painful—and potentially destructive—mode of healing. Surgical writers were acutely aware of the pain that their art caused. Accordingly, they often remind the audience of the need to consider the patient's comfort. The pioneering twelfth-century teacher and practitioner Roger of Parma states that the surgeon should create incisions "as tendurly and as delicatly as he may," while *The Lantern of Physicians*, an anonymous surgical text wrongly attributed to the London physician Roger Marshall, touchingly insists that prospective surgeons "schull make þe pacient ben in all softe & tranquyllyte boþ of herte and of bodye þat he may be inne."[64] Roger of Parma, who was especially sensitive to the difficulty of surgical treatment, administered different strengths of corrosive depending on the degree to which "the pacient be tendre and may not suffre it."[65] Many surgeons recognized this potential of their craft to replicate with the lancet the distorting effects of the wound itself. It is for this reason that Roger of Parma strictly prohibits experimentation with pharmaceuticals, which have potentially deadly effects, insisting that surgeons should use only those drugs that "worthi ffilosophures and leches haue ben expert in," and not "sley men with practysing of medicyns."[66] The thirteenth-century Italian surgeon William of Saliceto, Lanfranco's mentor, insists on the irreversibility of surgical accident when he solemnly cautions that the "þe sekenesse curable" is easily "turned to incurable by errour."[67] Indeed, the lack of a reliable anesthetic and a true means of staunching the flow of blood complicated medieval surgical treatment. A short treatise attributed to William of Touke instructs the surgeon to stop cutting at the point that "þe pacient falle for feblenesse or ellis meche bledyng."[68] William of Saliceto, citing the intense pain and hemorrhaging of incising the thigh, recommends eschewing this treatment altogether because "þis maner semeþ to me impossible and unable to be suffred of þe pacient."[69] One alternative to incision is the application of corrosive agents, the "potential cautery," to the afflicted area. William of Saliceto recommends substituting the potential for the actual cautery because sometimes "it is not possible to opne þe wounde of þe fistle with a rasour ouþer for drede of þe seeke or for þe makynge of þe membre."[70] To combat this "drede," surgeons developed clever strategies to help them maintain the patient's cooperation during such difficult treatments. We find in *The Lantern of Physicians* the recommendation of an intentional deception: "if þat hit be þat þe pacient bleede faste þe surgene must ordeyne þat þe pacient see nat his owne blood & telle hym þat he bledys nomore and telle hym þat if he bledde more þat hit were good and profytable to hym."[71] Another Englishman, the thirteenth-century physician Gilbertus Anglicus, endorses a similar technique. In administering corrosive chemicals to a wound, the practitioner should gradually acclimatize his patient: "bygyn with esy medycynes," writes Gilbertus, "and seyþe worch wyþ strengere."[72] We see, then, that surgeons often forego, to the best of their abilities, treatments involving incision if these are particularly troublesome for the patient, and they do everything in their power to alleviate the pain and fear involved in even the most minor surgical operations. That this aspect of the surgeon seldom finds expression in didactic religious literature demonstrates that religious writers were aware of the social power of metaphor to elicit the compliance of parishioners in Innocent's program of reform. Though the surgeon causes tremendous pain, he also heals the patient, an ambivalence of which confessors were very much aware. In invoking this metaphor, the confessor not only makes use of a common, and potentially terrifying, figure in his society, but encourages the internalization of a pained and wounded self-image. We can surmise that in viewing their bodies as wounded by sin, parishioners were more inclined to visit their confessor—indeed, their *spiritual surgeon*—for remedy. The medieval surgeon contended with these foreboding constructions while at the same time performing acts of healing that few others, including academic physicians, were capable of, and was therefore a figure both of punishment and forgiveness, damnation and salvation, fragmentation and redemption—in short, a figure that encapsulated the tensions inherent in late medieval piety in general, and therefore a figure of tremendous importance.[73]

Because the surgeon was both metaphorical and literal, I have divided this study into two parts. Part 1 examines poetic treatments of surgery as a metaphor for spiritual health, while part 2 comments on the effects such constructions had on the very men who embodied them: the priest who heals the wounds of sin and the surgeon who so frequently stood for him. The first two chapters of this study will therefore demonstrate the productive ambivalence of surgery, its unique ability to suggest the full range of Christian identities from sinful to virtuous, damned to saved, in two alliterative poems of the fourteenth century. Chapter 1 posits the religious poem *Cleanness* as an example of the surgeon as a metaphor for damnation, and of surgery as an instrument of divine vengeance. In recounting the Genesis episode of Sodom and Gomorrah, the *Pearl*-poet images the Dead Sea as an *anal fistula*, an important and controversial subject in nearly every surgical manual of the day. That the poet describes God's razing of these cities as both surgical and divine intervention demonstrates the profound influence that the types of metaphor articulated in confession exerted on the poetic imagination. By contrast, chapter 2 examines another poem of the fourteenth-century alliterative revival, *The Siege of Jerusalem*, to argue that the surgeon could stand not only for damnation but also for salvation, and surgery for the grace of God rather than His vengeance. Its protagonists, Titus and Vespasian, each receive two healings over the course of the poem, the first miraculous, the second surgical. In the first half of the poem, both men are spontaneously healed of their facial disfigurations the moment they accept the divinity of Christ, while in the second, earthly surgeons save the two from life-threatening wounds suffered in their vindictive siege of the Jewish city. The poet describes both recoveries in similarly salutary language, suggesting continuity between Christ's healing ministry and the secular craft of surgery. That *Cleanness* and *The Siege of Jerusalem* employ surgical metaphors to such vastly different effect is evidence of the extreme ambivalence through which this healing yet destructive craft could function so encompassingly as a metaphor for humanity's relationship with the divine.

The next two chapters illuminate the perspectives of the men who were made to embody this ambivalent rhetoric of spiritual health. Chapter 3 discusses the remarkable collection of penitential poetry by the Shropshire priest John Audelay, whose poems offer a unique glimpse into the psychology of post-Lateran Christianity from the perspective of one of its guardians. Audelay's increasingly blind, deaf, and diseased body rebels against the rhetorical commonplace that tribulation is merely a passage to clearer vision, fragmenting his identity in extremely telling ways. Chapter 4, by contrast, examines the fraught nature of embodiment from the perspective of the surgeon with reference to the Middle English version of John Arderne's *Practica*, a treatise that invokes the well-proportioned bodies of chivalric discourse as a means to disavow the fragmenting effects of the surgical operations it describes. Here I take a broad view of the related discourses of surgery and chivalry, showing their interdependence as disciplines that depend for their authority on the illusion of the body "whole and sound." Taken together, John Arderne and Audelay, just like the poets of *Cleanness* and *The Siege of Jerusalem*, reflect not only the broad scope of metaphors of surgery but also their power to both describe and directly affect the experience of being Christian in the fourteenth and fifteenth centuries.

PART I

SURGERY AND METAPHOR

CHAPTER 1

SURGERY AS DAMNATION IN *CLEANNESS*

The fourteenth-century homiletic poem *Cleanness* has at its core three Old Testament episodes: the Deluge (ll. 249–544), the destruction of Sodom (ll. 601–1048), and Belshazaar's Feast (ll.1056–1804).[1] This linear movement through sacred history is, however, interrupted after the second episode by a description of the Incarnation (ll. 1069–1108), which is depicted in language as flowery and reassuring as that of the three main episodes is grim and foreboding. This seeming arbitrariness of the poem's narrative structure has led some readers to suggest for it a unifying schema that emphasizes its potential as eschatology. Theresa Tinkle, for one, has described the poem's strategy as historiographic: "The homiletic move-ment gradually discloses the human need for and the divine offer of grace, roughly the progress of history from the Old to the New Testament."[2] For Tinkle, the poem presents history as a movement in which our "urgent need for divine salvation emerges more and more vividly."[3] Sarah Stanbury, arguing along similar lines, regards the poem as "an explication of an historical process, the developing and unfolding knowledge of God that culminates in the beatific vision, the sight of God on his throne."[4] Yet why, in so broad a historiographical exercise, does the poet concern him-self so rigorously with the corporeal, and especially with, as Allen Frantzen has put it, the "sights, sounds, and smells of Sodomy"?[5] I will argue that this emphasis on corporeality derives from a broader medical metaphorics, deployed by the poet to illustrate this progress of divine justice from Old Testament vengeance to New Testament grace. In this schema, sodomy, in its perceived status as "unnatural," serves as an appropriate sin with which to represent disease, while the grace of Christ, arriving with the Incarnation, is our "cure."

Cleanness, although nearly two centuries removed from the landmark events of the Fourth Lateran Council, reflects the council's influence in its use of medicine as metaphor. Pope Innocent was concerned to unite, under the rubric of a renewed orthodoxy, what he then believed was a splintered ecclesiastical community. Toward this end, Innocent attempted to distance the secular from the clerical, and he prohibited the clergy from engaging in "callings or business of a secular nature, especially those that are dishonourable."[6] He includes surgery, along with other duties involving bloodshed, in this grouping. Historians of medicine tend to overstate the scope of this edict; it was directed only at deacons, subdeacons, and priests and was less a condemnation of surgery than an attempt to tighten ecclesiastical strictures against the participation of the clergy in secular activity.[7] What this ruling did achieve, however, was the consolidation of a discursive division between surgery and medicine that had existed for centuries. Surgery was considered since Hippocrates to be the last resort, after diet and drugs, in a unified hierarchy of healing strategies. In the period following the Fourth Lateran Council, it is increasingly defined as separate from scholastic medicine, primarily by virtue of its status as handicraft.[8]

Around the time *Cleanness* was written, this discursive division had extended to the universities. As of 1350, the University of Paris required its medical graduates to swear a formal oath that they would never incorporate surgery into their practices.[9] Such changes to the medical infrastructure had the effect of, in the words of Carole Rawcliffe, "implicitly widening the gulf between theory and practice."[10] This gulf became so pronounced that the surgeon Jamerius, finding the scholastic environment increasingly hostile to his profession, complained of those who "find it below their dignity to know surgery or ridicule those who know it in front of their pupils."[11] *Cleanness* reflects this professional fragmentation by metaphorizing the Old and New Testament laws as contrasting medical treatments. The God of the Old Testament is presented imagistically as a surgeon who burns and severs the corrupt tissue from the social body. Realizing that surgery cannot heal the internal imbalances that cause such corruption, He sends Christ as the physic by which humanity may regulate its own health. *Cleanness* thus portrays surgical treatment as a potentially punitive treatment as compared to the more regulatory, preventative approach of the physician. The poet's fascination with medicine is not only confined to this eschatological progression, but it also, I will argue, permeates the explication of permissible sexuality as voiced by both God and Lot in the poem's controversial depiction of the razing of Sodom.

The poet's discursive interface of medicine with theology finds its most influential precedent in the Augustinian corpus. St. Augustine's indebtedness to ancient philosophical systems, especially Platonism, made him especially likely to merge the medical with the religious. Believing strongly in the Platonic notion of a divine order that underpins the sensible world, Augustine endorsed an ethical model in which behavior is governed by order and moderation, in keeping with the measure by which God governs all things. His well-known formulation that evil is itself insubstantial, but is in fact working in ways beyond our apprehension for our benefit, is only the most famous example of a philosophical enterprise concerned in large part with demonstrating the interdependence of seemingly contrarious elements.[12] Medicine, for Augustine, provides a convenient social example through which to demonstrate the pervasiveness of this ontological interdependence, since the body itself was governed by the interaction of separate and distinct elements. In *On Nature and Grace*, for example, Augustine writes that "it is quite possible for contraries not to be reciprocally opposed to each other, but rather by mutual action to temper health and render it good; just as, in our body, dryness and moisture, cold and heat— in the tempering of which altogether consists our bodily health."[13] This Galenic humoral model provides a fitting metaphor for the strained coexistence of the body and the soul, whose mutual contestation indicates not a flaw in Creation but a defect in the spiritual condition of humanity. Just as in medical theory the internal gathering of noxious humoral matter causes abscesses and swellings to appear on the skin, so too does excessively immoderate living beget what Augustine refers to, throughout his work, as "spiritual wounds" and "swellings of pride." In this fashion, Augustine analogizes sin as disease; and for every disease, there is need of a physician.

The Augustinian conceit of Christ the Physician is a familiar feature of medieval religious polemic, yet little has been done to explicate the broad scope of this complex metaphor. Augustine, throughout his work, displays knowledge of a wide array of healing practices that encompass not only the medical—drugs, salves, lifestyle, and the reading of pulses—but also the surgical, including binding, cautery, incision, amputation, and the application of corrosives.[14] In Augustine's time it fell to the physician to perform all these duties, and he clearly understands the role of the physician as inclusive. Within his broader metaphor, however, the surgical and medical branches of medicine serve different functions. Physic is used to connote conversion itself, while surgery is used to express the painful sacrifices that we must make in order to conform to Christ. In this schema, the Incarnation is literally the physic prescribed to us by God to bolster our spiritual health against the continuing repercussions of Original Sin. Humanity, writes Augustine, "was created at first faultless and without any sin; but that nature of man in which every one is born from Adam, now wants the physician, because it is not sound."[15] The Son is not only our physician but also our medicine and is often figured as an ointment or drug, an explicitly medical image that highlights the gentleness of *Christus Medicus* (Christ the physician). For example, Christ is thought to heal the spiritually blind just like "the eye-salve in the physician's hand."[16] Such gentleness contrasts with surgery, which Augustine uses to represent the more painful side of conforming to God, the trials that are sent us to temper our flesh and to teach us humility. Augustine depicts this figurative surgery as compassionate rather than cruel: "For that Physician is cruel who heareth a man, and spareth his wound and putrefaction."[17] *Cleanness* presents, in Augustinian fashion, a version of history in which humanity is figured collectively as just such a weakening patient. Because closest to Creation, Noah's ancestors were "the stalworthest that ever stod on fete" (l. 255). History is therefore the descent into ill health, a progress halted only with the Incarnation, when "ther was seknesse al sounde" (l. 1078). Yet, unlike Augustine, the poet develops his medical metaphor against a framework of temporal progression, a historiographical application made possible by the evolution of professional medicine into discernibly separate fields of practice.

In *Cleanness*, the episodes of the Flood and Sodom that precede the Incarnation are moments of crisis in spiritual health requiring surgical intervention. As we have seen, both spiritual and physical health is governed by naturally complementary components that, as a result of the Fall, have become imbalanced. It is therefore not surprising that in depicting pre-Incarnation humanity as profoundly unhealthy, the poet chooses to focus on sins that are against nature. Hence, the predeluvians "controeved agayn kynde contraré werkes" (l. 266), while the Sodomites "skyfted [God's] skyl and scorned natwre" (l. 709). Although it has recently been contended that the exceptional condemnation of sodomy in this poem indicates a specifically homophobic agenda, sodomy is also an appropriate metaphor for the imbalances that cause ill health. In guides to conduct such as the *Ancrene Wisse* and *The Book of Vices and Virtues*, sodomy is defined as belonging to the broader category of lechery, as its most severe form.[18] Lechery itself is generally defined as the failure of the individual to exercise sensual moderation. Indeed, St. Thomas Aquinas goes so far as to consider lechery "the paradigm type of immoderation,"[19] and from this we can infer that the sin of sodomy is paradigmatically immoderate. For Augustine, manifestations of such spiritual immoderation appear as swellings and abscesses, and these correspond to the literal wounds and ulcers that form from humoral imbalance. Similarly, the healthy characters in *Cleanness* are those who are enclosed, without openings, and these are contrasted with the amorphous crowds of sinners who symbolize the gathered corruption that forms lesions on the human body.

Such images of enclosure abound in the poem, and they serve to distinguish the spiritually unhealthy characters from the healthy ones. Noah encloses himself in a "cofer closed of tres clanly planed" (l. 310), while the goodness of Christ in the womb is evinced by how "he was clos there" (l. 1070). By contrast, the sinful predeluvians are depicted amorphously; they "dyyen al samen" (l. 400), while the Sodomites form "grete flokkes of folk" (l. 837). Noah and Lot, each accompanied by their children and their spouses, live measurably in contrast to the lecherous people around them. The most controversial scene in *Cleanness*—the confrontation between Lot and the Sodomites—is the clearest example of this dynamic. The Sodomites surround the enclosed structure of the Gatehouse and demand that Lot give up his visitors to their lusts. When Lot refuses, they attempt to find a way into his house, but "[t]hay lest of Lotes logging any lysoun to fynde" (l. 887). This "lysoun" can be seen as a distinctly corporeal image. The healthy body is often presented in medieval medical writings as enclosed, without lesions. The seventh-century etymologist Isidore of Seville defines the objective of medicine as the maintenance of this enclosed state: "In short, it includes every defense and fortification by which our body is kept [safe] from external attacks and accidents."[20] As Lynn Staley Johnson has observed, such enclosures are one of the *Cleanness*-poet's key devices of signification. The poem's protagonists are linked representationally to their enclosures in order to illustrate their roles as virtuous characters; Abraham, like his Oak tree, is paradigmatically paternal, and Lot, like his Gatehouse, rich and noble.[21] It is not only Lot's house, then, but also Lot himself who is without lesions.

Lesions, in the physiological sense, are openings in the flesh, and in the Middle Ages they were thought to signal the beginnings of an ulcerate wound. Ulcers feature prominently in medieval surgical writings—the external manifestation of internal, humoral corruption, it fell to the surgeon to excise such growths once drugs, diet, and purges proved ineffectual. Ulcers, then, are a fitting metaphor for the blemishes, caused by moral corruption, which must be excised from the soul. The following passage from the Middle English version of the *Cyrurgie of Guy de Chauliac* describes the process by which a defect of the humors manifests itself externally:

> The innatural humours ben voyded away and sente to dewe places for some manere helpynges, or þay be þrowen oute. . .of þe body, and þei gone wiþ þe blood. And sometyme þay beþ rotede, and þay maken feueres. And some ben þrowe out to þe skynne, and þay beþ resolued insensibly, or ellis sensibly (i. þat may be feled) by swetynge or by scabe or by bleynes or by aposteme.[22]

These wounds that appear "sensibly"—that is, externally—betray an internal, effluvial corruption, a physical analogue to the spiritual "spec of a spote" that the poet cautions will reveal us as sinners and exclude us from "the syghte of the Soverayn" (ll. 551, 552). Cleanness is therefore signified by a freedom from corruption both spiritual and physical, "Bothe withinne and withouten" (l. 20).

The linguistic similarities between vernacularized accounts of spiritual and physical corruption lend force to this view of Sodomy as an "innatural," pathological state. The poet uses the terms "kynde" (l. 697) and "agayn kynde" (l. 266) to denote permissible and impermissible sexual practices, a terminology derived from the penitential manuals that circulated in his day. For example, *The Book of Vices and Virtues* states that the priest, when hearing a confession to lechery, must establish "ʒif the synne be bi weye of kynde or aʒens kynde."[23] Surgical writings recast this moralistic dichotomy in a biological context and use the language of "kynde" to differentiate between natural and unnatural humoral fluids. Guy de Chauliac, for example, explains of humors that "some ben natural (i. kyndely)," while "some bene nouʒt natural (i. nouÿt kyndely)."[24] While the natural humors are used to nourish the organs of the body, the "innatural humours ben voyded away."[25] Humors that the body fails to expel through feces, urine, sweat, or the release of other fluids, need to be purged manually, either by bleeding or by enemas. John Arderne, for example, writes that "it auaileþ mich to hole men, constipate and noʒt constipate, if þai be purged twyse at lest or three or four tymeʒ in a ʒere," further enthusing that "þe benefite of it may no man noumbre."[26]

Just as the corrupt humoral matter that the body fails to assimilate is "voyded away," so too does the God of *Cleanness* act against the five cities with "a vengaunce violent that voyded thise places" (l. 1012). Such images of purgation are rich in this section of the poem. Words such as "voyded," "devoyded" (l. 908), and "upbrayded" (l. 848) all are used in relation to the Sodomites. God's vengeance is thus likened to a medicinal purgation, removing the harmful, "innatural" Sodomites before they can further infect the collective body of humanity. It is not uncommon to find in medieval moral discourse the likening of sodomy to disease, such as when the anonymous author of the *Ancrene Wisse* warns that simply mentioning it "muhte hurten alle wel itohene earen ant sulene cleane heorten." Indeed, states the *Ancrene Wisse*, one should, as with a disease, "swiðe flih þer frommard ear þu beo iattret."[27]

It is not surprising, then, to find that the treatment of ulcers in surgical writings develops a moral component. Surgeons, as a matter of course, advise wounded patients under their care to avoid immoderate sexual activity. We will recall that our anonymous London surgeon, writing in 1392, explains that immoderate activities, such as "leccherie," serve to "distempren þe body and meuen þe humouris, whos cours drawiþ to þe wounde & makiþ it empostime & discracen."[28] All surgical writers stressed the importance of the "non-naturals," external factors to health such as sleep, work, and copulation; immoderate use of these, or what Guy de Chauliac calls "malice of gouernance," was often seen as the cause of ulcers.[29] Moral intemperance not only creates "spiritual wounds," then, but also physical ones. That Lot is free from such lesions indicates his spiritual health; having lived in accordance with divine principles of order, he is without the abscesses, both spiritual and physical, that result from moral intemperance, and that, as we shall see, blemish the Sodomites.[30] As such, he is spared God's "cure," for as Augustine repeatedly states after Mathew 9:12, "They that be whole need not a physician, but they that are sick."[31]

This "cure" takes the form of the destruction of the five cities that follows, and the poet utilizes the vast descriptive opportunities such a scene affords by powerfully extending his medical metaphor. The poem's moral program is explicated throughout by a series of oppositions between purity and impurity, saved and unsaved; it is therefore crucial to the poem's symmetry that if Lot's purity be symbolized by his freedom from lesions, then the corruption of the Sodomites must be symbolized by a state of diseased ulceration. We must examine the poet's description of the Dead Sea in order to illustrate how this dynamic plays out in the poem:

> Blo, blubrande, and blak, unblythe to neghe,
> As a stynkande stanc that stryed synne,
> That ever of synne and of smach smart is to fele;
> Forthy the derk dede see hit is demed evermore.
>
> For hit dedes of dethe duren there yet;
> For hit is brod and bothemles, and bitter as the galle,
> And noght may lenge in that lake that any lyf beres,
> And alle the costes of kynde hit combres uchone.
> (ll. 1016–1024)

And, nine lines later,

> And as hit is corsed of kynde, and hit coostes als,
> The clay that clenges therby arn corsyes strong,
> As alum and alkaran, that angré arn bothe,
> Soufre sour and saundyver and other such mony;
>
> And ther waltes of that water, in waxlokes grete,
> The spumande aspaltoun that spyseres sellen.
> And suche is alle the soyle by that se halves,
> That fel fretes the flesch and festers bones.
> (ll. 1033–1040)

Allen Frantzen has already shown that the earlier speech of the Sodomites to Lot (ll. 842–48) abounds with anal puns; the poet equates the verbiage of the folk of Sodom with defecation.[32] In these lines, *asyse* refers to "arses," *segge3* to "sege," or "privy," and *briche* to "buttocks." Frantzen goes on to call the image of the Dead Sea "an anal image," but this time does not substantiate his description with linguistic evidence, presumably assuming an implicit continuity between these two passages relating to the Sodomites.[33] Closer attention to the imagery of the Dead Sea, however, reveals a similar use of the sort of bodily double entendres Frantzen identifies in the Sodomites' speech to Lot. These double entendres serve to extend the medical metaphor initiated in the description of the assault upon the Gatehouse. At the same time, the specific medical condition used to represent the Dead Sea substantiates Frantzen's claim that the image of the Sea is an anal one, rife with anti-Sodomitic implication.

It is necessary to begin at the end if we are to contextualize the lines quoted above—the remarkably animated description of the Dead Sea—within their broader metaphor. The Dead Sea, an unnatural place full of strange substances and death-like properties, is described pathologically. The use of the word "festers" in the final line of this passage is not simply a restatement of the Dead Sea's inimity to those "that any lyf beres" (l. 1023), but it is in fact punning on a well-known medical condition of the time. Festres, or *fistulae*, as they are interchangeably known, are a form of ulcer characterized by hardness of the surrounding flesh, terrible stench, and the wasting of the member.[34] The word "costes," as well, has a double meaning, signifying not only the coasts of the Dead Sea but also the more corporeal sense used in medical writings, such as when de Chauliac describes an ulcerated flank as a "coste of fistles."[35] The poet thus depicts a negative type of enclosure, one that contrasts radically with the architectural enclosures that, as Johnson has observed, link the protagonists to virtue. This dichotomy is established far in advance of this scene. During the previous episode, that of the Flood, the poet depicts God instructing Noah to build an Ark and of "uche clene comly kynde enclose seven makes" (l. 334), thus presenting an enclosure governed by the laws of nature. In this episode, the Sodomites, whose practices threaten the discontinuation of the species, do not internalize "kynde," but rather cast it out: the Dead Sea is "corsed of kynde, and hit coostes als" (l. 1033), and "the costes of kynde hit combres uchone" (l. 1024). The image is that of a body attacked on all sides by disease, a state caused by an overturning of natural balances from which the "clene" characters, in their enclosures, are immune.

Visually, the Dead Sea shares many traits with surgical accounts of a fistulate cavity. Where the Dead Sea is "[b]lo, blubrande, and blak," a fistulate opening may be known by its "hauynge wan and blo coloure, and derk."[36] The perpetual action from within the depths of the Dead Sea—its "waltes of water" and "spumande aspaltoun"—mirrors the movement of unnatural humors out of the fistula that, according to John Arderne, characterizes this condition: "And aftir auctours of cirurgie, a fistule is a depe aposteme... giffyng out quitour of diuerse colour and diuerse substaunce."[37] Ulcerate wounds were also often accompanied by an intense burning and aching. It is for this reason that Guy de Chauliac describes a particularly severe form of ulcer as *corrosium*, a "fretynge or gnawynge ulcer."[38] Like this ulcer, the Dead Sea "fretes the flesch and festres bones" (l. 1041) and contains "corsyes" (l. 1035). These corrosives of the Dead Sea are embedded in the "clay that clenges therby," just as, in surgical writings, fistulas were to be differentiated from other ulcers by "tho þinges þat cleuen substancially þeryn."[39] Lastly, the "stynkande stanc" of the Dead Sea parallels the horrible stench of a fistulate cancer, which de Chauliac claims is of "soche horrible attre and stinkynge þat it may nought be schewed by scripture."[40] This combination of linguistic punning and descriptive layering comprises a potent medical metaphor for the depth of the Sodomites' spiritual corruption.

At the same time as he figures the spiritual corruption of the Sodomites as a fistulate condition, the poet provides a correspondingly medical image of divine intervention. God acts surgically in destroying the Sodomites; the poet accesses a particularly painful yet increasingly prevalent mode of healing in his society to metaphorize the punitive, pre-Incarnation divinity. For all surgical writers, the cutting of fistula begins with a diagnostic to determine the depth of the corruption. Hence, in the beginning of the poem's second part we are told that God is a "gropande God" (l. 591), who, like a skilled confessor, can easily see the "venym and vylanye and the vycios fylthe" that is the cause of the Sodomites' downfall. In medieval medical terminology, the words "venym" and "fylthe" are used to describe two opposite poles on the scale of humoral corruption: the liquid humoral emissions from a wound, or "quitor," could be somewhat corrupt like venym, greatly corrupt like fylthe, or fall somewhere in between.[41] The severity of an ulcer could thus be determined sensibly. Having established by sight the signs of corruption—"I schal lyght into that led and loke myselven" (l. 691)—God decides eventually which course to take. To see the specific surgical tactics He employs, we must again turn to the description of the Dead Sea.

The Dead Sea is brimming with corrosive chemicals, chemicals that we have seen allude to the burning sensation that can make ulcers so painful. Yet these chemicals describe not only the condition but also its cure. They are itemized by the poet as "corsyes strong,/ As alum an alkaran, that angré arn bothe,/ Soufre sour and saundyver and other such mony" (ll. 1033–34). Also mentioned are "aspaltoun" (l. 1037), "pich" (l. 1008), and "brynston" (l. 967). *Mandeville's Travels*, the poet's source for the description of the Dead Sea, mentions that "[a]boute that see groweth moche alom and of alkatran."[42] Yet these details, in the source text, are nothing more than geographical markers, and they are innocently immersed within the opening details that place the Dead Sea near Jericho. In the poem *Cleanness*, these references to caustic materials are expanded and given prominence within the description of the Dead Sea itself. The poet recognizes their usefulness as extensions of his metaphorical fusion of surgical and divine intervention and thus transforms them into surgical details. All of the chemicals listed by the poet were commonly used in surgical practice to treat ulcerate wounds. Almost all are corrosives; that is, they are hot and dry in property, and they serve to burn away dead flesh.[43] The application of corrosives to a wound is called a "potential cautery," a chemical alternative to the "actual cautery," that is, burning with hot gold or iron.[44] The practice of cauterizing anal fistula seems for the Western world to have originated with the eleventh-century Arabic authority Albucasis, who regards it as the only plausible treatment for an otherwise incurable condition.[45] Anal fistula was, by the poet's time, so common an affliction that John Arderne, a contemporary of the poet, could make it a career specialty: "I helid many men of fistula in ano."[46] All surgical authors included a chapter specifically on this perilous affliction, and its frequency in medieval society lends a markedly corporeal bent to Frantzen's suggestion that the Dead Sea is an anal image. Although Frantzen makes this point with reference to other later medieval texts,[47] such an associative argument is hardly necessary: the proof of the Dead Sea's anality is contained within the very terms of its description. Just as the chemicals of the Dead Sea help to convey a specifically anal pathology, so too do they depict a corresponding cure.

Alum (l. 1035) was a key ingredient in the caustic mixtures used to cauterize anal fistula. A simple mineral derived from the alum-stone, alum could be burnt to form a powder or mixed with other chemicals and dissolved in water to create a compound substance.[48] John Arderne includes it in his recipe for *pulvis sine pari*, or "powder without peer," a medicine he employs against anal fistula because it "mortifieþ and bryngeþ out dede flesch or superflue or putred in al woundeʒ and vlcereʒ."[49] *Alkaran* (l. 1035) is another name for asphalt, which is listed subsequently under its more common nomination, *aspaltoun* (l. 1037). Asphalt is another substance used to treat ulcerate or fistulate conditions. Guy de Chauliac states, significantly, that "[a]spaltum is hardened scume þat is founden in þe Dede See," and that "it heleth vlcers."[50] The poet makes explicit the medical connotations of this "aspaltoun" by adding that it is of the sort "that spyseren [apothecaries] sellen" (l. 1038). That the poet restates the presence of asphalt after having already mentioned alkaran, and then signposts it as a medicinal substance, should alert us to the intentional invocation of a metaphorics relating specifically to surgical practice.

Soufre (l. 1036), or sulfur, sometimes called *brimstone* for its burning effects (literally, "burning stone"), is another substance the poet mentions that was used to dissolve mortified flesh. Albucasis recommends for anal fistula the application of "sulphur pounded with oil, until the place putrefies and the burnt tissue comes away in the pus."[51] Like asphalt, sulfur is alluded to elsewhere in this episode, once under the same name (l. 954), and once as *brynston* (l. 967). Next is *saundyuer*, a term used for glass gall,[52] which is listed by Lanfranco ("galle") in a recipe "for to slee a festre & a cancre."[53] The only substance listed that is not itself a corrosive is *pich*, or tar. Yet this too has its place in such treatment. Tar is often used as the adhesive in the making of "emplastres," (a clothy bandage) which is a method of applying medicinal substances to afflicted areas. Not only a medium by which to apply medicine, pich has its own healing properties. Arderne gives a recipe for an ointment "þat availeþ to cancrose vlcereȝ, and to wondeÿ, and to aposhemeȝ, of which floweþ out blode," and recommends it be administered in an "emplastre" with "blak pich, for pich haþe strenght or vertu of drawyng fro partieȝ bineþ to aboue."[54] That all these substances are used for the curing of fistulate conditions adds force to the image of the Dead Sea as a festering ulcer. More importantly, however, we can now see that the poet is using very specific medical details to metaphorize the pre-Incarnation God as "punitive" rather than "preventative." God acts surgically in destroying the Sodomites, who are depicted as a gathering of corrupt humoral matter on the collective body of Creation, and who therefore must be excised.

Immediately following this episode is the Incarnation, and the poet goes to great lengths to signal the transition to a period of grace: "For ther was seknesse al sounde that sarrest is halden, / And ther was rose reflayr where rote has ben ever, / And ther was solace and songe wher sorw has ay cryed" (ll. 1078–80). With the coming of Christ, sickness can be healed without the violence of surgery. Where God before had severed putrefied members of humanity, such putrefaction can be transformed with Christ. Where "rote has ben ever," there is now the potential for salvation rather than extermination. The detail here is carefully chosen to create an oppositional symmetry between these two scenes that frame the birth of Christ. "Rote," the conventional term for the putrefaction of wounded flesh, is in surgical writings most commonly associated with an ulcer: "A filthy and a roten wounde is called an vlcer."[55] In this fashion, the poet extends the representation of spiritual corruption as a physical ailment beyond the previous scene of Old Testament punishment, to the merciful New Testament present.

Yet the poet carries over not only the medical metaphor of the disease, but of the cure as well. With brilliant economy, he opposes not only "rote" with "rose reflayr," but he also opposes "rose reflayr" with the corrosives depicted in the previous scene. Roses, like the chemicals listed in the Dead Sea, feature prominently in the medieval antidotary. Unlike the chemicals of the Dead Sea, however, roses are not "corrosive," but "confortatyue";[56]

where corrosives "bursteþ or brekeþ and brenneþ þe skyn,"[57] oil of roses and other comfortatives "swageþ and softeneþ þe brennyng & þe prikkyng, þe smertyng and þe akyng."[58] The presence of music at the bedside scene of Mary's labors is also another indication that a new, gentler physic has replaced the violence of surgery. There is now "songe wher sorwe has ay cryed" (l. 1080), played upon organs, pipes, and viols (ll. 1081–82). In the poet's time, music was believed to act as a healing agent, a humoral restorative whose harmonious properties could reverse the imbalances that are the cause of illness. As John Trevisa argues, "by swete voys and song[es] and armonye, acoord, and musik, sike men and mad and frenetik comeþ ofte to hire witt aÿee and hele of body."[59] A powerful healing agent, music was also thought to enhance the post-operative healing of surgical wounds.[60] We see in these lines, then, a clear opposition between pain and comfort, an opposition that the poet affects through his strategic positioning of specific medical details.

Christ, in a manner described by the poet as "clanner then any crafte cowde devyse" (l. 1100), goes on to cure victims of dropsy and leprosy, as well as the blind, lame, and feverish. When healing, Christ "fonded he never / Nauther to cout ne to kerve wyth knyf ne with egge" (l. 1103–1104). Indeed, His incisions are so gentle and precise that not "alle the toles of Tolowse moght tyght hit to kerve" (l. 1108). Christ, as the arbiter of grace, has no need of the cauterizing agents employed before the Incarnation, or of the "toles" of incision and burning that mark a treatment as surgical.[61] Andrew and Waldron have argued that the poet did not intend to refer to Toulouse here, but must instead have meant "Toledo," which was known for its production of knives.[62] Yet Toulouse was certainly known for surgery. De Chauliac places "Tholose" first in a list of cities where in his day "were Cirurgiens wirkynge."[63] Also, John Arderne smugly tells us of a patient whom he managed to cure, but who had come to him only after exhausting the resources of "lecheȝ and cirurgienȝ" in several cities, including "Tolows,"s well as in "many other places" apparently not worthy of mention.[64] The poet's choice of Toulouse might therefore be intentional, and meant to signal the redundancy of the tools of surgical "crafte" in this new era of grace. The context of this passage—the breaking of bread at Emmaus—can easily accommodate so corporeal a detail, since transubstantiation, for the faithful, transforms bread into the literal body of Christ. Christ's coming allows for the curing of the causes of disease, not just the symptoms; He is Himself the medicine, transmitted through the Host at Mass, a ceremony the poet alludes to in the poem's opening lines (ll. 10–15). The beginning of post-Incarnation history thus is marked by a change in the way God relates to His Creation. This change is metaphorized by the distinction between surgery and medicine, a distinction made possible by the historical circumstances as regards the medical infrastructure of the poet's time.

If the first two sections of the poem are meant to show the transition in divine healing from the surgical to the medicinal, then the third and final episode inverts this metaphor altogether. Centering on Belshazaar's mistreatment of the vessels of Solomon's temple, this section returns to the theme stated in the poem's opening lines: the need for purity among those who "hondel ther his aune body. . .and prestes arn called" (l. 8). The surgical metaphor is therefore seen to work both ways: not only are we handled by a "gropande" God, but we too "grope" His body. The grace of Incarnation brings with it certain responsibilities, and the anxiety that Christ's literal body in the form of the Host might be misused surfaces in much penitential literature. The poem thus is strewn with both negative and positive examples of hands and handling: the protagonists make proper use of their hands, the antagonists improper. Christ possesses "gropyng so goud" (l. 1102), while God rebukes Sarah for doubting "my hondes to work" (l. 663). Noah uses handicraft in accordance with God's will that he "make to the a mancioun" (l. 309), while Belshazaar, against God's will, "false fantummes of fendes formed with handes"(l. 1341).

Robert Blanch and Julian Wasserman have called Christ's healing hands a "perplexing symbol" in the poem,[65] yet the poet's obsession with manual imagery can be seen as an extension of the surgical ethos that I have argued is evident throughout. The importance of hands to surgical discourse cannot be overstated. The etymology of surgery, literally "handicraft," becomes the basis by which all surgical authors describe their profession. De Chauliac repeatedly calls it a "manuel craft."[66] Even those authorities who insist on surgery as a science, such as the late-thirteenth-century Italian teacher and practitioner Lanfranco, define it largely as a manual discipline: "he that wole knowe what siurgie is, he moot vndirstonde, þat it is a medicinal science, which techiþ us to worche wiþ handis in mannes bodi."[67] So, surgeons stressed the importance of clean hands. According to John Arderne, for example, a surgeon should have "clene handes and wele shapen naileÿ and clensed fro all blaknes and filthe."[68] Early historians of medicine took this as Arderne's prefiguring of surgical hygiene,[69] but this emphasis on cleanness possesses a deeper, spiritual import. Because the body represents the artisanship of God, it must be handled reverently. Craft therefore figures largely in the poem as a proper mode by which to relate to the divine. Indeed, the poet warns us that we will not be admitted to heaven with "handes unwaschen" (l. 34). As we will see in the following chapter, this relationship between the mechanical arts and Christ's salutary grace allows the surgeon to represent not only damnation but salvation as well.

Solomon, who made the holy vessels that Belshazaar will abuse, stands in the poem as a paragon of such proper, "clene," handling. The similarities between the descriptions of Solomon, the Incarnation, and heterosexual intercourse (as voiced by God and Lot) alert us to another way in which surgical craft operates in the poem: as a metaphor for procreation. During the episode of the Incarnation, the poet describes God's act of immaculate conception as so "comely a kest" (l. 1070). Reproduction is therefore depicted as a craft that God employs to effect a pivotal moment in sacred history. Thus, in the poem, embryology and divinity are rhetorically intertwined. Solomon too performs a "kest," crafting the vessels in accordance with God's teachings. He employs "the syence that hym sende the soverayn lorde" (l. 1454), in order that he may "compas and kest" (l. 1455) the vessels that shall honor Him. In this period, "syence," or *scientia*, was the term used to describe the teaching of surgery, while the performance of surgery was considered craft.[70] God, who teaches Solomon to create the vessels, engages in another *scientia* when He teaches the Sodomites the "craft" of procreative intercourse: "I compast hem a kynde crafte and kende hit hem derne, and amed hit in myn ordnaunce oddely dere" (ll. 697–98). With this conscious repetition of key words, the poet links conventional craftsmanship—that of ornamental or functional objects—with procreation. God thus is seen to teach the craft of Creation, in language reminiscent of the relationship between a master craftsman and his apprentice. The poet was arguably thinking of surgery in particular when composing this conceit—the French surgeon Henri de Mondeville provides a similar comparison when he writes that "God himself practised as a surgeon when He made the first man out of clay, and from his ribs made Eve; and. . .decided to honour all surgeons by performing with his own hands the office of a surgeon."[71]

Lot duplicates this same metaphorical register in his offer to teach the wicked Sodomites a more efficacious form of copulation: "Bot I schalle kenne yow by kynde a crafte that is better" (l. 865). Such a restatement of so specific a conceit serves to make clear the poet's intention that we link craft with procreation. This metaphorizing of heterosexual intercourse as craft complicates recent readings of the poem that have taken its absence of a clear procreative imperative as evidence that the poet constructs a homophobia based on aesthetics.[72] Craft is always bound up with teleology. As a Middle English version of Henri de Mondeville puts it, "bothe surgian and euery othir craftiman that wole worche by rule and reason, he muste ȝeue his entent to a certeyn entencioun outhir to a certeyn ende."[73] That the poet employs this register of craft to suggest the superiority of procreative sexual intercourse is hardly surprising. By the poet's time, there is a well-developed tradition in medical theory to describe the act of conception in distinctly craft-like terms. This tradition begins with Aristotle, who uses the example of carpentry to describe the process by which the passive, female matter is shaped into a fetus by the formal male principle: "it is the shape and form which pass from the carpenter, and thus come into being by means of the movement in the maternal."[74] Subsequent theorists are attracted to this formulation that posits the male semen as the sole formal principle in reproduction, a model that by the poet's time had almost entirely replaced Galen's more inclusive schema of two contributing seeds.[75] The Pseudo-Albertus Magnus, a contemporary of the *Cleanness*-poet, uses a similar metaphor in his *De Secretis Mulierum* (*Women's Secrets*) to illustrate the dominance of the male seed in the process of conception: "For just as a carpenter is the efficient cause, and the house is the effect,. . .so the male seed alters the female menses into the form of a human being."[76] Just a few lines earlier, he states that the female substance is worked on by the male spirit, "as a smith fashions with a hammer."[77]

The poet, then, is representing procreation as craft in accordance with an ancient medical tradition, and surgery, defined as a craft, is compatible with such a representation. These scenes, however, suggest an even deeper indebtedness to medical knowledge. Popular embryology, when set along-side conventional religion as an influence on the poet's construction of sexuality, problematizes the view that the poet's praise of heterosexuality is a subversive literary act motivated by a dogged determination to condemn same-sex intercourse. In a recent, eloquent monograph, Elizabeth Keiser argues that the poem uniquely prefigures contemporary modes of homophobia by expressing revulsion at same-sex intercourse based not on modality but on aesthetics. According to Keiser, "*Cleanness* astonishes not by its harsh denunciation of same-sex love, but by its divergence from the procreative and patriarchal logic of compulsory heterosexuality as natural order."[78] If the poet is departing from convention, however, it is not a dis-cursive departure, but, rather, a descriptive one. While the conventional limits on the description of sexuality, both homo- and heterosexual, are undoubtedly exceeded in this poem, the praising of sexuality itself can be seen to resemble traditional medical discourses that took pleasure as a necessary component of the procreative process. The remainder of this chapter will reassess the scenes where Lot and God praise heterosexuality, in order to show that their perceived, puzzlingly vitriolic instances of misogyny and heterosexism are in fact best understood as echoing contemporary episte-mological commonplaces regarding the reproduction of the species.

One such troubling instance concerns Lot's treatment of his daughters. Lot, after stating that he will teach the Sodomites "a crafte that is better," offers to them his daughters as an alternative to their non-procreative sexual practices. In the process, he engages in an impromptu sales pitch: "Hit arn ronk, hit arn rype, and redy to manne" (l. 869). This line has been the source of much modern critical indignation, in no small part because its shocking commodification of the women seems to exceed the requirements of the narrative context. As Michael Calabrese and Eric Eliason have stated, "No matter how many times one reads this passage it is difficult to suppress feelings of revulsion at Lot's description of his daughters, which almost intolerably amplifies the biblical text."[79] But these lines, I believe, are less jarring (if, to us, no less distasteful) when placed in their proper context of medieval reproductive theory. The passivity of Lot's daughters—as material to be worked upon by the Sodomites as they, the Sodomites, learn the "kynde crafte" of procreation—is an appropriate figuring of what, in the poet's time, was almost always seen as a process in which the active male dominates the passive female. Indeed, investigations into the differences between the sexes frequently made use of the book of Genesis to demonstrate that female subjection, because ordained by God, is inscribed directly into the physiology of women. Hildegard of Bingen, for example, argued that women are physically inferior due to their secondary status in the order of Creation, while Thomas Aquinas claimed that female births result from the imperfect operation of the male reproductive power, accidents of nature that ensure the propogation of the species in our fallen world.[80] John Trevisa summarizes succinctly this Aristotelian model of female passivity: "In the male beþ vertues formal and of schapinge and werchinge, and in þe femel material, suffringe, and passiue."[81] Not only general scholastic texts but surgical ones as well took this model as axiomatic. Thus we find Guy de Chauliac depicting the womb in agricultural terms, as "þe felde of mannes generacioun."[82] Lot's invitation to the Sodomites is figured in similarly agricultural terms: his daughters are fertile fields, "ronk," "ripe," and "redy to manne." The extent to which we may see the poet's description of the daughters as evidence of a personal or disproportionate misogyny is therefore mitigated by his obvious—indeed, his inescapable—participation in a historically and culturally specific mode of biological description.

God's praise of procreation, like Lot's, suggests the language of embryological theory. In this controversial passage, God proclaims that lovers "moght honestly ayther other welde, / At a stylle stollen steven unstered wyth syght" (ll. 705–706). Far from condemning the passion of intercourse, God, in the most colorful terms, endorses the pleasure to be derived from it: "Luf-lowe hem bytwene lasched so hote / That alle the meschefes on mold moght hit not sleke" (ll. 707–708). Calabrese and Eliason have argued that this passage is astonishing because its "defense of sexuality ignores procreation," and is thus at odds with a theological tradition that judges all sexual acts "by their consonance or dissonance with this principle."[83] The poet thus facilitates his praise of heterosexuality by establishing what they call "a new sexual order based on pleasure."[84] This reading is, however, misleading in its presentation of God's praise of heterosexuality as a radical divergence from medieval discursive orthodoxy. Indeed, this passage is well within the discursive limits of a conservative medical tradition that contributed much to the medieval construction of the body, and which contains within its very terms a procreative imperative. In scholastic discussions of human reproduction, the procreative function was thought to inhere in pleasure itself. The copulative process, far from being the stuff of damnation, was often seen in such discussions as the ultimate example of divine creativity. The eleventh-century monk, medical authority, and prolific translator, Constantinus Africanus, explains,

> The Creator, who wanted the race of animals to continue firmly and stably, planned for it to be renewed by intercourse and generation, so that by this complete renewal the race would not perish. He therefore gave animals suitable natural members for this specific function; and he put in them such an admirable virtue and sweet pleasure that all animals are overcome with delight in intercourse—for if they disliked it, their race would surely perish.[85]

In this formulation, the pleasure of intercourse is intertwined with the capacity for reproduction. Furthermore, God is seen to endorse this pleasure, which He gave us to ensure the continuity of the species. *Cleanness* is very much within this tradition, presenting a God who not only teaches us the "kynde crafte" of procreation, but who also privileges this sexual capacity as an especially "dere" component of His "ordenaunce" (l. 699). Keiser's argument—that *Cleanness* "represents a religious endorsement of loveplay that is nothing short of astonishing to the medieval period"[86]—is therefore tenable only if we read the poem as religiously monodiscursive.

This view of sexual pleasure as divinely ordained was so pervasive that surgeons, who often strove to tailor their writings to the medical mainstream by incorporating into them general biological knowledge, frequently espoused it. Thus Lanfranco, in his discussion of the anatomy of the male genitalia, states that God designed intercourse "so þat generacioun miȝte be multiplied wiþ greet delite."[87] In order for generation to occur, a reasonable amount of heat had to be present in the reproductive organs to effect the transformation of blood into sperm. God's assertion that the heat between lovers "lasched so hote" does not describe simply an ardor of sexual passion, as both Keiser and Calabrese and Eliason take it,[88] but also suggests the innate heat that the body produces in order to create generative material. Lanfranco lists such heat as another component, along with pleasure, of God's plan for the continuity of the species: "he knewe þat a man schulde be maad of moist substaunce, as of sperme, in which natural hete schal worche."[89] God's endorsement of sexual pleasure is therefore not so radical when seen dialogically with medical constructions of the sexual experience, which take as inseparable pleasure and procreation. That the presence of a procreative imperative is only implicit in God's speech does not indicate a strategic absence of teleology from the scene, but suggests the extent to which the poet assumes reproduction to inhere within the very terms of his discourse.

In *Cleanness*, medical discourses function for the poet as a means by which to connect his often unpleasant, sometimes ethereal religious polemic to issues of sickness and health, everyday realities that, in an age ravaged by plague, bloodshed, and starvation, would have had universal significance for the poet's contemporaries. This poem must be seen as but one example of the medieval artist coming to terms with elusive, spiritual concepts by linking them to the pervasive and animating context of an always precarious physical welfare. I therefore hope to have shown with this chapter not only the importance to *Cleanness* of discourses outside the conventionally religious, but by extension the necessity of seeking out the discursive polysemy that resides necessarily in every medieval text beneath the vast, seemingly impenetrable surface of Christian orthodoxy. Medicine, in *Cleanness*, is a metaphor both for the mutual interaction between deity and humanity, and also for the responsibility of moral choice, a position of salutary agency that is, for the poet, the legacy of the post-Incarnation era.

Yet surgical markings were not always associated with the negative application of this agency, as punishment through divine retribution; indeed, the surgeon could also be a figure of salvation, and surgical inscription on the body a sign of holiness rather than depravity. When we turn to compare the representation of surgery in *Cleanness* to that of *The Siege of Jerusalem*, it becomes clear that, because of this productive ambivalence, the figure of the surgeon could uniquely encompass the many tensions inherent in late medieval piety.

CHAPTER 2

SALVATION AND *THE SIEGE OF JERUSALEM*

Introduction

In their classic study into the phenomenon of body image, Seymour Fisher and Sidney E. Cleveland describe selfhood as the maintenance of an identity distinct from the outside world, achieved through the development and perpetuation of firm phantasmic barriers at the limits of the body. Their clinical findings help shed light on the surprising bodily emphasis of religious poems such as *Cleanness*, which dwell on the corporeal as the means to address larger, more spiritual concerns. In interviewing patients, Fisher and Cleveland found that individuals with weakened senses of self-worth constantly made reference to images of mutilation, wounds, and incisions, while those with firm ego boundaries tended toward images of armor, enclosures, and other protective surfaces. As we have seen, *Cleanness* describes damnation as a gaping, leaking, surgical wound, and starkly contrasts this with the enclosed, protected bodies of the saved. In their data from patient testimonials, Fisher and Cleveland uncovered a startlingly similar set of images, which they grouped under the category of "openings in the earth that have no set boundaries."[1] Patients with unhealthy ego boundaries, when shown random shapes, frequently saw both a "bottomless abyss" and a "geyser spurting out of the ground";[2] significantly, both these images are part of the *Cleanness*-poet's depiction of the Dead Sea.

The fourteenth-century alliterative poem *The Siege of Jerusalem* represents the other side of the surgical metaphor. In this poem, surgical treatment brings about the saved, enclosed body, rather than the damned, perforated one. It associates the surgeon not with the punishment of damnation but with the dissemination of God's grace. In this way, the *Siege*-poet proceeds on the same principle as *Cleanness*, but makes the opposite use of the vast range of meaning that the ambivalent status of the surgeon affords him. While *Cleanness* presents a surgical image equating sin with an open wound, and surgery with the punishment of damnation, *The Siege of Jerusalem* presents the surgeon's treatment as thoroughly healing, connecting it to God's own salutary power. In this sense, *The Siege* makes use of surgical imagery to reassure, rather than terrify, its Christian audience.

The Siege of Jerusalem is suffused with medical matter, including leprosy, fevers, and, of course, wounds. Indeed, the very structure of the poem revolves around four distinct yet related healings. These, in turn, are divided into two sets of episodes, involving Titus and Vespasian as the recipients. The first healings are religious in nature, and they involve the conversion of these two central characters to Christianity. The second occur during the action of the siege itself and describe the ministrations of medical personnel. Although these second healings are presented as secular, they are in their very terminology linked to the earlier, miraculous recuperations and constitute similar instances of divine intervention. Interestingly, the poet goes to great lengths to ensure that these latter healings are understood as surgical: a "leche" tends to Vespasian's wounded foot, while Titus is cured by a man who "surgyan was noble."[3] Unlike in *Cleanness*, however, surgery is depicted as neither punitive nor painful; for the *Siege*-poet, surgery is an extension of the grace and mercy of God, an application of the *Christus Medicus* metaphor undiluted by an Old Testament ethos of justice. As we shall see, *The Siege of Jerusalem*, for all its blustering representations of violence, maintains its focus squarely upon the salvation of the Romans rather than the damnation of the Jews. Where *Cleanness* might be said to polemically target the sinners who are among its audience, *The Siege of Jerusalem* seems intended more for the saved. These two poems, then, are concerned with opposite sides of Christianity's moral divide. That surgery is the central metaphor for each is a significant illustration of the polysemy that attended later medieval attitudes toward surgeons and their unique mode of medical treatment.

It could be argued that the surgeon was a common enough presence on the late medieval battlefield, and the two episodes involving surgery were nothing more than chivalric details of the sort common to romance descriptions of warfare. Yet there is another, related structural component in the poem. The repeated invocation of Christ's Passion suggests that we are meant to view these two sets of healing episodes as part of a single, extended discourse on the continuing need for God's grace in the poet's time. The Passion not only opens the poem but also establishes its theological context. Implicit in Christ's wounded body is its resurrected counterpart, a transformation that not only prefigures but also enables the bodily wholeness that all faithful and properly confessed Christians will enjoy at

Judgment Day. This image occurs twice in the poem, first at the beginning and then again in the middle. The latter instance stands between the two healings, the miraculous and the surgical, implicitly unifying them. The depictions of healing thus assume the force of parable and are meant to remind the audience of the rewards of sustained religious observance.

As Caroline Bynum has so influentially documented, the later Middle Ages saw a tremendous amount of debate centered on resurrection, and especially on the particulars of corporeal reassembly. Although the accounts of bodies in the afterlife varied immensely in their details, the theological principle was unchanging: that, in Bynum's words, "Christ's resurrected body is the paradigm for ours," and "wholeness—non-partibility and non-passibility—is God's ultimate promise to mankind."[4] In connecting the wholeness promised through God's grace with that effected through surgical treatment, the poet posits surgery as a metaphor for nothing less than salvation, and especially for the bodily intactness that the saved will enjoy in the afterlife. This chapter will use *The Siege of Jerusalem* to show that surgery could stand not only for punishment, as it does in *Cleanness*, but also for grace; not only for fragmentation, but also for redemption; for the fortification of Christian identity, not merely for its failure.

Although we saw in the last chapter that the surgeon can serve as a metaphor for God, it may nonetheless seem surprising that I would posit surgery as a metaphor for salvation. Medievalists have become accustomed to descriptions of the surgeon's discursive position in medieval society as polluted, a debased intruder into the sacred enclosure of the body. Marie-Christine Pouchelle, in her landmark study of the thirteenth-century Montpellier surgeon Henri de Mondeville, established the medieval surgeon as a figure of remarkable ambivalence. Indeed, surgeons could be learned scholars or illiterate operators; favored courtiers or obscure barbers; respected practitioners or conniving charlatans. However, according to Pouchelle it is his association with blood that most contributed to the social debasement of the medieval surgeon. Successive ecclesiastical rulings had expressed concern over priests who perform surgery with their hands and then, thus polluted, go on to handle the sacraments. Pouchelle locates this taboo ultimately in Leviticus and shows how its legacy was felt in regulations governing the profession of butchery, the prohibitions concerning magical rites, and the controversies over anatomical dissection.[5] It is his similar contact with the enclosed matter of the body that rendered the medieval surgeon socially problematic. According to Pouchelle,

> The surgeon, then, was a man of blood. Polluted. Like anyone who infringes a taboo and is affected by the forces enclosed in the taboo object, he was

both affected and impure. This is to a large extent why his contemporaries found him so disquieting.[6]

Although Pouchelle's broader analysis does take into account the ambivalence of the surgeon rather than merely his negative associations, the above statement has, in isolation, become nearly axiomatic as regards the role of the surgeon in medieval society. Thus Bynum, in discussing the various social practices thought to threaten both the integrity of the body and its ability to reassemble in the afterlife, associates the surgical profession with fragmentation rather than redemption. Surgery, "because it severed flesh," meant a partitioning of the body that even torturers were required to stop short of.[7] Because the promise of material continuity was thought to be essential to religious identity, any practice threatening the integrity of the body in life was associated with corporeal fragmentation, the punishment of the damned. For Bynum, then, the surgical body joins the embalmed body, the leprous body, and the divided saint's body as a specter of fragmentation, of the forfeiture of that bodily wholeness that Christ guarantees is the reward of the saved.

There is another reason why the potential of the surgeon to signify salvation has gone relatively unnoticed. As we saw in the last chapter, the surgeon was socially inferior to the scholastic physician, whose priestly background made him a more obvious symbol of Christian grace than the guild-oriented barber-surgeon. This is certainly true of *Cleanness*, in which Christ practices a gentle *physic* as compared to God's harsher, surgical approach to His pre-Incarnation subjects. In the early Middle Ages, monks practiced all three branches of medicine—diet, drugs, and surgery—as a unified hierarchy of healing strategies. Two main factors can be said to have precipitated the subsequent division of medicine into the surgical and the medical professions: the growth of the universities and the rulings of the Fourth Lateran Council. Eager to see their profession represented in university syllabi, physicians strove to establish the art of medicine as philosophy, a science based on universal, unchanging principles. A major obstacle to validating medicine in this fashion, however, was its unavoidable focus on the body, which was considered a profoundly mutable and ignoble entity. Another obstacle was the manual nature of much medical practice, including the performance of surgery and the concoction of drugs. By the thirteenth century, scholastic physicians found that they could maintain their status "only by abandoning to specialists of lower social standing the two aspects of the discipline that demanded use of the hand: surgery and pharmacy."[8] The Fourth Lateran Council of 1215, meanwhile, prohibited higher orders of clergy from practicing surgery. In this new medical economy, physicians continued to be ordained as priests, whereas the practice of surgery was left to clergy in lower orders or to the ranks of laymen. As Carole Rawcliffe has argued, "the confessor and the physician were often the same person" and occupied a lofty role in society as compared to the surgeon, who was seen to engage in an "*ars mechanica* (the mechanical arts), a practical, hands-on activity."[9] A dichotomy thus develops by the later Middle Ages in which the physician is associated with philosophical truth and spirituality, and the surgeon with bodily matter and the mechanical arts. Given this accepted historical picture, it is no wonder that scholars tend to regard the medieval surgeon as a locus of extreme anxiety.

Yet at the same time as the surgeon could be said to have occupied an inferior social position to his physician colleagues, there was also a well-developed theological tradition that did not denigrate, but rather vaunted the mechanical arts—and, with them, surgery—as an important component in the divine plan for salvation. Although it can be argued that a theological tradition, no matter how positive, could not offset the material reality of the mechanical arts as servile, it must be stressed that this tradition is in fact an integral component of Neoplatonist, and therefore Christian, thought. The notion of God as an artisan, and of Creation as the product, permeates patristic writings, and the continuing tensions inherent in this formulation reflect the tensions of Christianity in its infancy as it strove to accommodate ancient polytheistic systems. From this concept of an artisanal God comes the related notion that in emulating such craftsmanship, we ourselves can return to some semblance of the divine likeness in which we were created. In this chapter, I intend briefly to trace the history of this metaphor that connects the mechanical arts to the operation of God's grace, and then to show that the Augustinian origins of *The Siege of Jerusalem* make this poem especially likely to access this tradition. I will also argue that surgery would have been a particularly visible craft in North Yorkshire where the poem was composed, and that its markedly corporeal character lends itself to the salvationary aesthetics that so powerfully underlie the action of *The Siege of Jerusalem*.

Surgery as Salvation: The Intellectual Tradition

By the fourteenth century, Aristotle had assumed such high stature in the minds of philosophers and theologians that he was known simply as "The Philosopher." Yet Plato's influence was equally important in forming Christian thought throughout most of the Middle Ages. Plato's account of the creation of the world, as preserved in his dialogue *Timaeus*, would have a profound influence on Christian scriptural exegesis. In this account, the figure of the artisan—an image culled from Greek agrarian society and equally resonant for Plato's medieval successors—looms large both as a metaphor for and description of the divine intelligence. Having reasoned that all objects that comprise the world must by necessity have originated with some ordering principle, Plato posits a demiurge who, in perfect charity, "desired that all things should approach as near as possible to being like himself."[10] To this end, the demiurge fashioned the world after the model of the artisan. The artisan, for his inspiration, looks not to transient objects but to unchanging principles, the eternal models that presuppose all things in the sensible world:

> Again, everything that becomes must of necessity do so by the agency of some cause; without a cause nothing can come to be. Whenever the maker of an object looks to that which is always unchanging and uses as model of that kind in fashioning the form and quality of his work, all that he thus accomplishes must be good.[11]

Because the world is good, and all good is based on the eternal rather than the mutable, it must therefore have been created by a perfect intelligence that could perceive in full the world of Forms, the conceptual templates to which all matter should conform. Because the sensible world is only a copy, however, it resembles the divine only inasmuch as a product approximates the will and intention of its artificer. If the demiurge is nothing less than an artisan, ingeniously constructing objects from ideal exemplars, he is also nothing more: the demiurge, like the artisan, is bound both by the autonomous world of Forms and by the materials available from which to fashion their likeness. This image of the artisan would prove problematic for Christian theologians, whose conception of the divine was predicated upon an absolute and unassailable quality of omnipotence. As we shall see, Plato's concept of a God who works from existing blueprints, and with existing materials, proved hard to reconcile with the Christian concept of a deity with whom nothing may be coeternal.

The Platonic notion of a divine artisan who works from design continued to influence pagan thinkers throughout the early Christian era. In particular, the rising tide of skepticism in pagan intellectual circles was met repeatedly with the argument that the complexity of the sensible world could only be the result of a deliberate and magnanimous act of artisanship. Increasingly, Plato's demiurge would be described as Nature itself, a concept that, though often expressed pantheistically, comes to resemble more and more the singular Judeo-Christian God. In an argument Christian theologians and scholars became fond of repeating,[12] Cicero, debating with the cynical Academics, held up the human body as the ultimate proof of the folly of disbelief: "what artisan other than nature, whose cleverness nothing can surpass, could have demonstrated such great ingenuity with the creation of the senses?"[13] For Cicero, the artisan metaphor is not limited to the action of Creation itself, but pertains equally to the objects of divine productivity available for our contemplation—that is, the sensible world. Our heads are "citadels," and our eyelids "ramparts";[14] the body itself is crafted on the principles of architecture, a testament to the order and design of Nature. As we shall see, such architectural imagery figures prominently in *The Siege of Jerusalem*.

More importantly, however, there is in Cicero some suggestion of the emanationist philosophy that was transforming Platonic thought in these early centuries of Christianity. The products of divine creation, because they emanate from a perfect being that is not itself created, are therefore of a lower order than their originator. Nature, however, provides us with a number of gifts with which we may better approximate divine perfection. One of these provisions is the human capacity for manual labor, a gift that enables us to edify ourselves with painting, sculpture, and music, and also to feed, clothe, and house ourselves, not to mention construct temples and magnificent cities.[15] The gifts of intelligence also allow us to engage in astronomy, which, because it brings knowledge of the gods, leads to religious devotion and a corresponding sense of justice and morality.[16] Through these gifts, we can achieve "the blessed life which is equivalent and analogous to that enjoyed by the gods."[17] Galen too argues that among all living creatures, man is alone in being "godlike," and that to "compensate for the nakedness of his body, he received hands, and for his soul's lack of skill, reason, by means of which he has arms and guards his body in every way and equips his soul with all the arts."[18] This pattern of return, of restoration to the glory of what Plotinus called the "One," would feature strongly in Christian discussions of salvation throughout the Middle Ages, and it would carry with it a discourse of artisanship that counteracted, at least rhetorically, the servile position of the mechanical arts in medieval conceptions of the social order.

The Early Church Fathers frequently adopted the design argument found in Cicero and in Galen, replacing the encompassing yet vague concept of Nature with that of the monolithic Christian God. As in Cicero, the sensible world retains its function as an object of contemplation through which to better appreciate the divine creativity. In the fourth century, St. Ambrose, in his *Hexameron*, Christianizes the pagan image of the artisan:

> There are other arts of such a nature that, even when the processes of oper-
> ation cease, the handiwork remains visible. As an example of this we have
> buildings or woven material which, even when the artisan is silent, still
> exhibit his skill, so that testimony is presented of the artisan's own work. In
> a similar way, this work is a distinctive mark of divine majesty from which
> the wisdom of God is made manifest.[19]

While Ambrose has little trouble transposing this Platonic notion to a Christian setting, he does not confront the tensions that reside in the margins of this passage. Early Christian theologians eager to find in the authority of Plato a validation of the New Testament encountered two major difficulties. First, Plato's demiurge, while not created, fashions the world from materials already extant, and therefore blasphemously coeternal with the divine. Second, the Forms from which he creates are not of his own devising, but they exist autonomously in some ethereal yet undisclosed location. These factors place unacceptable limits on God's power, compromising his status as the absolute Creator.

It is ultimately St. Augustine of Hippo who unflinchingly confronts the legacy of Plato and illustrates the ways in which Platonic philosophy did and did not lend itself to a staunchly monotheistic religious system. When St. Augustine, in his commentary on Genesis, comes to compose his own artisan conceit, it is with a more combative spirit than his contemporary St. Ambrose. Taking as his proof the "harmonious unity" of living bodies, Augustine insists that all beings exhibit the work of "God their artisan," whose methods follow the divine principles of "measures, numbers, and order."[20] Augustine finds it necessary to qualify this metaphor in order to defend it against those who would prefer to retain Plato's vision of a less-than-omnipotent demiurge:

> And, therefore, we correctly believe that God made all things from nothing. For, though all formed things were made from this matter, this matter itself was still made from absolutely nothing. For we should not be like those who do not believe that Almighty God could have made something from nothing, when they observe that carpenters or any workmen cannot produce anything unless they have something out of which to make it. For wood helps the carpenter, and silver helps the silversmith, and gold the goldsmith, and clay helps the potter so that they are able to accomplish their works. For if they are not helped by that matter out of which they make something, they cannot make anything since they do not themselves make the matter. A carpenter does not make wood, but makes something out of wood, and the case is the same with all the rest of these workmen as well. But Almighty God did not have to be helped by anything that he had not made so that he could make what he wanted. For if something that he had not made helped him to make those things he wanted to make, he was not almighty, and that is sacrilegious to believe.[21]

Although Himself a "workman," God's creative power is in no way constrained by the variables that bind the earthly artisan to a circumscribed range of possibilities. In this way, Augustine is able to employ a metaphor with tremendous resonance to an increasingly agrarian society, but without having to compromise the quality of ultimate transcendence upon which the Christian conception of God depends. This is Plato's demiurge taken to its logical conclusion, its defining schema of unity to plurality unfettered by a vague and irreconcilable notion of things that exist coeternally with the divine.

Even more important than his liberation of the artisan metaphor from its secular limitations, however, is Augustine's emphasis on the role of grace. As previously suggested, the pagan model of the divine artisan participates in an emanationist schematics, in which the various provisions for our return to perfection are taken for granted as part of the natural circularity through which all material beings are eventually restored as Form. For Augustine, such gifts cannot be taken for granted. Because of the pernicious legacy of the Fall, the body disintegrates throughout life. It is only through God's grace that it is restored at Judgment Day: "after that death which we all owe because of the bond of sin, we must believe and hope that the body will be entirely changed for the better at the time of resurrection."[22] For Augustine, grace allows for some partial movement back toward the perfection of the prelapsarian era, an earthly foreshadowing of the restoration granted in the afterlife. To this end, God bestowed upon us the capacity for reason and, by extension, "all the important arts discovered and developed by human genius."[23] In listing these arts, Augustine follows his pagan predecessors and includes medicine, architecture, weaponry, and various other crafts that aid us in our disadvantaged state. However, in this new Christian schema these arts are not ours by right, but they must be exercised without ever forgetting the debt of devotion that we owe to our divine benefactor. For Augustine, then, the mechanical arts are at once both divine and servile, spiritual and earthly, an ambivalence mitigated only by our own discernment. Used properly, crafts represent "assistance to God in His works"; like all things in Augustine's moral universe, they must be applied in moderation "so that we do not devote ourselves to them."[24] The theology of Augustine, as it pertains to the artisan metaphor, represents a movement from the conditional to the transcendent, and in its attitudes to the mechanical arts, a movement from right to privilege. These formulations would prove highly influential for subsequent theologians attempting to find a place for the mechanical arts in the categories of knowledge.

In composing his *De diversis artibus* (On the Diverse Arts), the eleventh-century Benedictine monk Theophilus Presbyter, a skilled metallurgist, strove against the snobbery of his monastic peers. The Benedictines had increasingly viewed manual labor as unworthy of both themselves and their fellow religious.[25] The view that the mechanical arts should be servile to contemplation, a prejudice that had dogged even Augustine, is in

Theophilus met with the assurance that, though we once used craft knowledge immoderately, we have now "transmitted it in every part to the predestined age of Christian religion."[26] Theophilus's argument is simple but remarkable: humanity, because created in the image of God, inherited the divine capacity for artisanship, for which the paradigm is Creation itself. Although the Fall deprived us of immortality, forcing us to live in a state of relative deprivation, our situation is improved somewhat by the gifts of wisdom and intelligence, which allow the diligent among us to "attain a capacity for all arts and skills, as if by hereditary right."[27] This is a remarkable conflation of two key ideas we have seen so far: God Himself as artisan, and the arts as salutary emanations of God's wisdom. Theophilus, then, gives evidence of a changing attitude toward the mechanical arts, one that does not merely permit them a place in religious activity, but recognizes their unique resemblance to the Divine Will.

This change in attitude to the mechanical arts culminates with the *Didascalicon* of Hugh of St. Victor, whose specific validation of craft knowledge will be taken up by later thinkers such as Bernardus Silvestris and Bonaventure. Hugh, who was German by birth, lived and wrote at the Augustinian abbey of St. Victor in Paris. The School of St. Victor was an important center for Neoplatonic thought. Its founder, William of Champeaux, is best known for his firm support for the existence of universals, or "realism," in which he was opposed by a burgeoning school of Aristotelian "nominalists" that included his own star pupil, Abelard.[28] As Martin Thornton notes, the "Augustinian-Platonic thought indigenous to St Victor" became so associated with Victorine theologians that "this strain of spirituality is to be called not Augustinian but Victorine, and the English fourteenth century is to become saturated with its spirit."[29] The Victorines, like all Augustinian thinkers, engaged in a sort of mysticism tempered by the spirit of rational enquiry. In true Platonic fashion, Hugh considered each individual part of Creation to be the visible expression of an idea originating in the mind of God, a Christian rendering of Plato's theory of Forms. The contemplation of the natural world therefore leads to the "true knowledge of God, not just a general sense of wonder at his harmonious works."[30] Because of its high investment in such realist doctrine, Victorine thought would play an important role in the survival of that particular Platonic rhetoric that vaunted the mechanical arts.

Although writing in the early twelfth century, Hugh of St. Victor seems uninfluenced by the renewed interest in Aristotle that was sweeping the universities of Europe. The *Didascalicon* is a thoroughly Augustinian and Neoplatonic exposition on the place of secular knowledge in the divine plan for salvation. In the fifth century, the Roman senator Cassiodorus had boldly attempted to reconcile secular learning with the contemplation of the divine, positing an "unbroken line of Divine Scriptures and the compendious knowledge of secular letters."[31] Following Cassiodorus, Hugh divides philosophy into four parts: theoretical, practical, mechanical, and logical. Among the mechanical, Hugh includes fabric making, armament, commerce, agriculture, hunting, theatrics, and medicine. Because these arts take their inspiration from nature, they are called "adulterate"— not purely spiritual, they depend upon the exertions of the human artisan.[32] Yet the gift of Wisdom, the ability to contemplate divine truths, encompasses a wide range of activities that effect the "restoring of our nature's integrity, or the relieving of those weaknesses to which our present life lies subject."[33] Just as humans are patterned after the Divine Idea, so too do the "products of artificers" imitate nature and "express the form of their exemplar."[34] Thus the weaver fashions clothes on the model of the furry animal; the armorer imitates the shell of the turtle; and the architect looks to the mountains in constructing a domed lodging.[35] This inclusive vision of philosophy must have been very attractive to the majority of Christian laymen, because it posits the active life as an important component of salvation.

It is here that we see surgical medicine achieve its tenuous place in the scheme of salvation. Hugh lists surgery among these arts and defines it as "cutting, sewing, burning," and "setting and joining."[36] Vincent of Beauvais, as translated by Caxton, is less charitable regarding the status of surgery, arguing that only those disciplines that directly contemplate divine truths can participate in the liberation of the soul, because "the sowle ought to be liberal as thyng that is of noble beyng, as she that cometh of God, and to God wille and ought retorne."[37] Yet clearly for Hugh, the mechanical arts *do* return the soul to God: the four categories of the arts are not autonomous but continuous; the mechanical is simply the execution of the theoretical and participates equally in the descending order of gifts provided by Wisdom.[38] The surgeon, then, can play a prominent role in salvation, returning the body to its prelapsarian state while at the same time providing a valuable link between the corporeal and the spiritual, the religious and the secular.

The twelfth and thirteenth centuries saw a marked increase in the influence of Aristotle, precipitated by the rediscovery of his scientific works through the translations undertaken by Gerard of Cremona and others working at Toledo. Aristotle viewed Platonic Forms as, at best, metaphors for rational forethought, and he denied their actual existence: "the Form," writes Aristotle, "is useless to the sciences."[39] Aristotle argues that there can be no single idea across the different sciences, because many ideas exist even within a single category. Within particular sciences, the doctrine of Forms is seen as equally useless: a doctor does not consider health but the health of human beings, and a particular human being at that.[40] Because Aristotle dismisses the notion that knowledge unilaterally serves the purpose of restoring humanity to the likeness of a single idea, he necessarily relegates craft knowledge to an extremely servile position. Whereas philosophy must observe unchanging principles in nature, the artisan is not concerned "with things that are by nature, since these have their origin in themselves."[41] Deprived of its place in the common pursuit of a singular divine knowledge, the mechanical arts become detached from any higher aim.[42]

The Victorine justification of craft knowledge was so popular, however, that it survived the Aristotelian renaissance. As Aristotle's influence increased, propagated by nominalist theologians such as Albertus Magnus, Robert Kilwardby, and Thomas Aquinas, his privileging of empirical observation often fused with the more mystical approach of the Victorines.[43] The mid-twelfth-century Chartrian writer Bernardus Silvestris, despite his obvious interest in the "new science," retains a strong Platonic element in his writings on the categories of knowledge. In his commentaries on Virgil's *Aeneid*, Silvestris divides philosophy into four parts, including mechanics, "the knowledge of human works connected with corporeal needs."[44] Although these arts are adulterate, they nonetheless join wisdom, eloquence, and poetics in "bearing light" against the darkness of our fallen natures. One of these arts is surgery, "medicine which uses cauterizing, incision, and other manual operations."[45] The mechanical arts would prove no less important for the towering thirteenth-century Franciscan theologian Bonaventure, whose avowed Aristotelianism is hardly in evidence when he describes knowledge as a descending order of "lights" with their "origin in one light."[46] Explicitly following Hugh, Bonaventure describes "the light of mechanical art" as less bright than theory, yet still a vital component of knowledge.[47] As M-D. Chenu astutely points out, this image of light in medieval theology was not merely a literary conceit, but it was "the consistent effort of the metaphysics of emanation, which saw not only intelligences but nature itself as filled with the light of the supreme and motionless One and as becoming assimilated to the One through conscious or unconscious contemplation of it."[48] Bonaventure too lists surgery among those arts that help restore us in God's image, defining it as "the amputation of members."[49]

We see, then, that the centuries leading up to *The Siege of Jerusalem* established a theological tradition that elevates the mechanical arts—works of the hand—to salvationary status, roughly the status of philosophy itself. These writers define medicine inclusively, placing both surgery and physic within the category of the mechanical. However, as Danielle Jacquart has noted this theological tradition does not accurately reflect the reality of medieval medicine and its status in the universities. By the twelfth century, the division between surgery and physic, the animating principle of *Cleanness*, was already very much in evidence. While medieval surgery may confidently be said to belong to the *ars mechanica*, physic, which involves the less invasive treatments of diet and drugs, was by this time gaining a higher status than it had ever before experienced. The Salernitan masters, working in the eleventh century, had fought hard to establish their discipline as a science. Their translations of Galen and other Greco-Roman and Arabic authorities had rendered untenable the view that medicine is entirely divorced from the speculative sciences. The *Didascalicon* of Hugh of St. Victor therefore exhibits "clear indications of a reluctance to accept the development of scientific medicine."[50]

Surgery, by contrast, was by this time wedged securely into the category of the mechanical arts. Only in Italy was surgical training available at the university level.[51] Elsewhere, it was in the control of guilds and undertaken by apprenticeship. To be sure, there were learned surgical treatises, those written by university-educated men who could claim thorough and encompassing knowledge of both the theoretical and practical sides of medicine.[52] Yet these were the exceptions, and to take them as indicative of the state of the surgical profession in the fourteenth century would be highly misleading. Even these learned surgeons tended to acknowledge their associations with the mechanical arts. In the fourteenth and fifteenth centuries, in the wake of the Fourth Lateran Council, a number of surgical treatises were translated into Middle English, making available to non-Latinate practitioners the works of such authorities as William of Saliceto, Lanfranco, Theodoric of Cervia, Guy de Chauliac, John Arderne, and others. The result was that even comparatively unlearned practitioners "learned to participate in essentially the same system of medical ideas as their Latinate colleagues."[53] In the eleventh century, Avicenna had posited theoretical knowledge as indispensable to the practicing physician, who "should take the fundamentals as granted and desist from asking for any proof of their existence."[54] By the late thirteenth century, surgeons could make this same claim to theory. Lanfranco, for example, insists that the surgeon should learn "fisik, þat he mowe wiþ good rulis his surgerie defende."[55] Yet the prominence of the vernacular manuals by no means divested the surgeon of his associations with craft. From these treatises, we get a sense of a discipline aware of its status as a mechanical art, yet simultaneously eager to subvert that very position. A Middle English version of the surgery of Theodoric of Cervia advises its audience that although surgery, "handwarke on the bodie," is the "last instrument of medicine," it is also indispensable as that without which medicine "mowe not remeve the evil of the bodie."[56] Theodoric further endorses surgery as prestigious by alluding to "Galien and oþer olde surgeans,"[57] and this despite Galen's rather equivocal views on the value of surgical treatment.[58] Similarly, an anonymous author of a brief surgical treatise begins by stating that one has "recours to the surgien" for such mundane afflictions as "apostmes," "vlcers," and "peynes of bones," but then goes on to establish his academic knowledge by discussing the nonnaturals and other matters of medical theory.[59] No sooner has our anonymous author launched on this academic trajectory than he derails it with a statement perhaps more in the spirit of protest than deference: "thise thyngs perten more to this lordis the phisicianes and surgyens ben nat called in hem but for manuell worchings."[60]

Regardless of the insecurity with which some practitioners described their art, most surgeons were proud of their practical and efficacious roles. Throughout the Middle Ages, surgeons would strenuously defend the mechanical character of their discipline. Our anonymous London surgeon admonishes those practitioners whose academic pretensions cause them to balk at performing such common manual operations as phlebotomy: "ffor it is a surgians craft to lete blood, þouʒ we for oure pride haue left it vn-to barbouris. ffor Galien & Rasis as her bokis beriþ witnes, diden it wiþ her owne hondis."[61] The fourteenth-century priest John of Mirfield, though not a surgeon himself, authored a surgical treatise in which he laments the division between physicians and surgeons, letting the blame fall squarely upon the former:

> In ancient times, unless I err, it was the province of physicians to practise surgery, to shave and to bleed. But today a great distinction is made between surgery and medicine. And this, I believe, stems from arrogance because they [physicians] disdain working with their hands. But more than this, I think it is because they have learned nothing of the method of operating which is the proper business of all physicians.[62]

Many surgeons believed that this "method of operating" was as much a mental exercise as a physical one. The court-employed fifteenth-century English surgeon Thomas Morstede, like John of Mirfield, was disillusioned with the surgical profession in his day, complaining that "now adays ar many surgens of name but not of dede."[63] In his Middle English surgery derived from the Latin *Philomena* of the prosperous London surgeon John Bradmore,[64] Morstede defines the surgeon not only as a "craftyous man,"[65] but also as one whose manual exertions are grounded in rigorous a priori knowledge. Partaking in a common analogy, Morstede insists that the surgeon, when cutting, must be able to envision the various muscles and sinews beneath the flesh just as a carpenter must be able to see the proportions of the wood upon which he works.[66] Morstede argues that the word "anathomie" refers literally to "a ryght devydynge and determenynge of mannis body" and, in a clever play on words, claims that this act of "devydynge" is also the "entent of all surgery."[67] This movement from the epistemological to the anatomical sense of "devydynge" amounts to a similar conflation of Form and product as that which, as we have seen, defined the Neoplatonic theology of craft and associated the artisan with divine creativity. Henri de Mondeville made this association explicit by arguing that God "practised as a surgeon" when He fashioned Adam, "and again when from the dust He made a plaster with which He rubbed the eyes of the blind man and so restored his sight."[68] For Henri de Mondeville, the surgeon's association with craft rendered him not merely equal but rather superior to his physician colleagues, whose tasks of judging urine and reading pulses do not resemble divine creativity in the slightest.[69] We see, then, that surgery, because a mechanical art, could partake of a theological tradition in which crafts do not prevent but rather contribute to the restoration of perfection, and therefore to salvation itself. Indeed, it is precisely because surgery is so tied to the body that it can rise above its servile position, that it can uniquely signify not only the act of Creation, but also that promise, that central article of faith—indeed, that very telos of Christian worship—that at Judgment Day the pious will be restored in body and relieved of all deformity and disease.

Surgery and the Austin Canons

Although *The Siege of Jerusalem* has received little critical attention, several fine studies have appeared within the last decade that attempt to make sense of this astonishingly violent poem by examining it in its historical context. Elisa Narin Van Court, finding that the few critics who have written on the poem tend to regard it as an example of unrestrained anti-Semitism, identifies a clear rhetoric of toleration amidst the constant bloodshed. In place of a "straightforward and brutal poetic," Narin Van Court sees a "sympathetic narrative strand," evidenced by the Roman sympathy for the besieged Jews and the poem's surprising absence of pejorative terminology.[70] Because of its unusual tolerance, Narin Van Court speculates that *The Siege of Jerusalem* is the product of an Austin Canon, whose adherence to Augustine's writings would have exposed him to "the doctrine of relative toleration."[71] This doctrine is, as Narin Van Court explains it, "a theological formula in which the Jews are accorded a role in Christendom: alive, but in servitude; alive, but socially and economically degraded; alive, but as symbols of Christ's Passion."[72] Taking into account the poem's Yorkshire provenance, as well as the quality of humane moderation that characterizes both *The Siege of Jerusalem* and the Rule of St. Augustine, Narin Van Court suggests Bolton Priory as a possible point of origin.[73]

While Narin Van Court was preparing her article, another one appeared that comes to the same conclusion, albeit through a very different methodology. Ralph Hanna III is rather less charitable to the anonymous poet; while he does admire the poem's undeniable moments of beauty, he also labels it "stridently anti-semitic."[74] Having examined the eight manuscripts of *The Siege of Jerusalem* in their monastic contexts, Hanna comes to the conclusion that Bolton Priory was most likely the poet's home; in addition to linguistic evidence, he finds that Bolton's library contained several of the poet's learned sources, as well as numerous vernacular poems, including *The Siege of Jerusalem* itself.[75] Linguistic and codicological evidence aside, it is ironic that another reason Hanna regards Yorkshire as an appropriate location is because of its "noxious" history of anti-Judaism, and most infamously at York in the twelfth and thirteenth centuries—in other words, for exactly the opposite reason that Narin Van Court favors the same locale.[76] This points to the strength of the Augustinian influence in the fourteenth century, in that *The Siege of Jerusalem* retains a tolerant spirit in an age "when the doctrine of toleration had almost entirely yielded to a more hostile ideological and practical treatment of the Jews."[77] The Augustinians preserved, however, not only an unfashionable doctrine of tolerance toward Jews but also an increasingly antiquated view of the mechanical arts as salutary rather than merely mundane.

By the fourteenth century, the Aristotelian schematization of knowledge, in which the mechanical arts are seen as an unfortunate necessity, had achieved prominence. Although the elevation of craft undertaken by Hugh of St. Victor and others retained its influence in later medieval discussions of the mechanical arts, "the effort to upgrade the educational status of the *artes mechanicae* was abortive."[78] For many thinkers of the fourteenth century, the emphasis was no longer on the role of craft in aiding salvation, but it was on "how crafts functioned as adjuncts to the various sciences."[79] In this intellectual context, surgery could hardly suggest the transcendent. On the contrary, it would seem that the surgeon must become even more aligned with the mundane, while his physician colleagues remain unaffected in their social status. Yet the intellectual activities of the Austin Canons remained indebted to the Neoplatonic trajectory established by such early houses as that at St. Victor. Victorine and Chartrian texts were heavily represented in Augustinian libraries, as were those of St. Augustine himself.[80] Furthermore, Augustinian houses proliferated rapidly from the end of the eleventh century. By the time of the dissolution of the monasteries under Henry VIII, nearly two hundred and fifty houses of Augustinian canons had been founded in England alone, more than for any other order.[81] This meant that the fairly conservative theology of the Augustinians would retain some prominence in the later Middle Ages.

The Austin Canons were formed in response to the growing need for an alternative to the strictness of the Benedictine Rule, and especially to the

Cistercian demand for renewed fidelity to that Benedictine Rule.[82] Secular clergy, their attention newly drawn to the problems inherent in the monastic model, began to see possibilities for the circumscription of their own communities. These clergy, mostly clerks in large church dioceses, had long since abandoned the apostolic life; now, in the early twelfth century, it seemed possible for them to unite under what would turn out to be a comparatively permissive Augustinian Rule.[83] The Rule of St. Augustine is derived from a document known as Letter 211, one of Augustine's letters of advice to a community of female religious.[84] More a paean to communal values than a proper rule, the Rule of St. Augustine allows for tremendous flexibility in terms of conduct, and could therefore accommodate a wide range of communities. If this flexibility helped ensure the rapid growth of the Augustinians,[85] it also meant that they would be the object of much disdain from the more traditionally monastic Benedictines and Cistercians.[86] Eventually, however, the "prestige of St Augustine's name" overrode all objections, and by the mid-twelfth century Augustine was regarded as a monastic legislator of equal importance to Benedict.[87] The Augustinians themselves helped to propagate this prestige. Adam of St. Victor, the abbey's famed liturgical poet, praised "Father Augustine" as "the one Faith's strength and stay," whose "holy rule" leads its followers to "their fatherland of light."[88] In claiming for their own the single most dominant figure in Christian theology, the Austin Canons obtained the reputation, as J.C. Dickinson put it, "of the highest sanctity."[89] By the fourteenth century, the Austin Canons were held in so high a regard that Chaucer, in *The Canon's Yeoman's Tale*, felt that he had to preface his portrayal of a corrupt Augustinian alchemist by assuring "worshipful canons religious" that he is targeting a single bad example, and does not mean to "sclaundre youre hous."[90] This statement, we might add, appears to contain none of the complicating ironies that Jill Mann identified in Chaucer's "anti-clerical" portraits of the Monk and Friar.[91]

The Austin Canons not only retained a theology of the mechanical arts as salutary, but lived by a Augustinian Rule that invokes the practice of surgery as a central metaphor. The Canons were permitted to engage in a number of mechanical arts, so long as they were of benefit to the community. *The Bridlington Dialogue*, a twelfth-century commentary on the Benedictine Rule by a Yorkshireman known only as "Robert the Scribe," states that, although an Austin Canon should primarily serve God, there are "many occupations which are needful for the monastic life."[92] Among these, Robert includes fabric making and agriculture, two of the seven mechanical arts identified by Hugh in his *Didascalicon*. Hugh himself identifies a third art in his own commentary on the Benedictine Rule, whereby "it is our duty to seek medicines for the ills of the body, in order that we may produce fruit in God's service."[93] Furthermore, the Austin Canons were involved heavily in the establishment and maintenance of hospitals. The largest hospital in medieval England, St. Leonard's at York, was Augustinian, and even those hospitals not established by Austin Canons still tended to follow the Rule of St. Augustine.[94] That surgeons operated charitably in these institutions seems clear from a variety of sources, including the stipulation in the will of the wealthy fifteenth-century mercer Jon Don that the surgeon Thomas Thornton "contynewe in his daily besynes and comfort of the poure, sore and seke people" who require treatment "in the hospitalles of Seint Mary, Saint Bartholomewe, Saint Thomas, Newgate, Ludgate and in other places whereas peple shal have nede."[95] The aforementioned John of Mirfield was closely associated with both the Austin Priory of "Saint Bartholomewe" in Smithfield, London, and also the nearby hospital. John of Mirfield wrote two Latin encyclopedias: the first, *Florarium Bartholomei*, contains a single chapter on medicine amidst a miscellany of religious subjects, while the second, the *Breviarium Bartholomei*, devotes itself entirely to medical theory and practice.[96] As Faye Getz has noticed, this division of topics suggests "the dual nature of his association" with both priory and hospital, a conflation of spiritual and physical health that can be said to characterize not only John of Mirfield's own preoccupations but also those of the Augustinian order as a whole.[97] This is not to suggest that other orders did not have sophisticated surgical provision; Benedictine houses were employing phlebotomists, barbers, and master surgeons by the thirteenth century.[98] It does seem clear, however, that surgery was an important part of the monastic life as defined in the Augustinian context.

The Augustinian Rule invokes medicine not only in the practical sense, but also participates in the Augustinian tradition of Christ the Physician. The notion of *Christus Medicus* provided theologians, sermonizers, and poets with an engaging and quotidian apparatus with which to convey elusive spiritual truths. As we saw in *Cleanness*, poets often image Christ as a surgeon who has come to heal a wound or a physician with salves to cure the feverish and the blind. Augustine is widely credited with shaping this metaphor into the form it would assume throughout the Middle Ages.[99] The Augustinian Rule turns on a similar motif; its followers are "no longer slaves under the law," but "a people living in freedom under grace."[100] The belief that the Son has come to save humanity from sin is the central tenet of Christianity, and also the very foundation of *Christus Medicus*. We should therefore not be surprised to find in the Rule the related metaphor of the "wounds of sin." In encouraging brethren to enforce appropriate codes of conduct, Augustine resorts to an explicitly surgical metaphor:

Do not consider yourselves unkind
when you point out such faults. Quite the contrary,

you are not without fault yourselves
when you permit your brothers to perish
because of your silence.
Were you to point out their misdeeds,
correction would at least be possible.
If your brother had a bodily wound
which he wished to conceal for fear of surgery,
would not your silence be cruel
and your disclosure merciful?
Your obligation to reveal the matter
is, therefore, all the greater
in order to stem the more harmful infection of the heart.[101]

This language of pathology—of wounds and "infection"—is identical to the language used in Augustine's other, more well-known formulations of the "wounds of sin,"[102] and it is meant to connect the familiar figure of the surgeon to Christ's salutary power. This passage can also be read, however, as evidence of the presence of surgical treatment within Augustinian communities. As noted before, the Rule of St. Augustine is markedly humane as compared to the more exacting one of St. Benedict. Nowhere in the Rule of St. Augustine is this quality better illustrated than in its generous provisions for medical treatment. Regardless of whether or not his condition is visible, a brother complaining of sickness must be taken seriously, and a remedy should be sent for.[103] If there is concern that the monk is requesting a particular treatment—for instance, a medicinal bath—for pleasure rather than genuine need, the brothers must consult a physician to settle the matter.[104] By contrast, the Benedictine Rule makes no such allowance for the importing of secular physicians.[105] Hugh of St. Victor, in an example of the relative laxity of the fourth-century Rule of St. Augustine coming into conflict with the stricter, post-Gregorian mindset, expressed anxiety that monks might exploit this provision to obtain some respite from their religious and communal obligations.[106] The presence of surgery is evidenced not by those brothers who desire to make gratuitous use of their medical privileges, however, but by those who are afraid to be treated at all. Augustine insists that every brother submit to proper medical care, and, if unwilling to comply, "shall do what has to be done for his health."[107] If we read this edict as continuous with the earlier, surgical metaphor, then the reticence of these brothers can be seen to relate to the presence of surgical treatment within Augustinian houses.

We are now prepared to rejoin the fourteenth century and the question of surgery in *The Siege of Jerusalem*. Surgeons governed the medical profession in North Yorkshire, where *The Siege of Jerusalem* was probably written. Phillip Stell, in an excellent survey, outlines the progress of the healing profession in medieval York.[108] According to Stell, not a single practitioner in York can be shown to have graduated from a university. From 1301, all medical practitioners had to be examined by the municipal authorities and were required to demonstrate enough proficiency in minor surgical operations that they could at least treat wounds. Because of this premium on wound treatment, the barbers and barber-surgeons of York drastically outnumbered physicians by the mid-fourteenth century. As Stell notes, a common theory as to why barbers began performing surgery relates to the Fourth Lateran Council. Barbers, it is argued, were called to cut the tonsures of the monks and, because of their manual dexterity, came to assist in monastic surgical operations. When canon law forbade monks from practicing surgery, the barbers took over. Barbers were considered artisans, and they were organized as a craft union. By the fifteenth century, their guild was responsible for the evaluation and supervision not only of surgeons working within the city, but also physicians. If any of these barbers had assisted monks in nearby Augustinian abbeys, they could well have acquired an excellent education in surgery. The Austin Canons valued secular learning, and the Rule of St. Augustine provided for an hour to be scheduled each day in which monks could borrow manuscripts.[109] Their collections contained many of the authoritative surgical treatises of the day, including those of Roger of Parma, John Arderne, Lanfranco, and Guy de Chauliac.[110] The *Siege*-poet, if indeed an Austin Canon, could easily have acquired surgical knowledge through these means, and may well have associated this knowledge not with servile crafts but with salvationary grace. It now remains to examine the ways in which he uses this knowledge in the service of literary expression.

Surgery as Salvation: *The Siege of Jerusalem*

When it is discussed, *The Siege of Jerusalem* is, as we have seen, generally the object of a certain critical dismay. Despite the poem's lush ornamental flourishes and sumptuous descriptions of late medieval warfare, critics have seemed for the most part unable to divert their gaze from its extremely violent narrative foreground, and with good reason: the terrible events of the last century have ensured that any such extended, and seemingly gleeful, description of genocide against Jews is to be met with an unavoidably outraged response. Upon first reading this underappreciated work, one is indeed struck not only by the sheer frequency with which Jewish bodies are torn, pierced, mutilated, and dismembered by the avenging Romans, but also by the lengths to which the poet has gone to describe such violent exertions in their every gory detail. That the poet takes such apparent delight in describing this violence has led Derek Pearsall to bemoan his "crude and narrow vindictiveness."[111] The poet's amplification of this violence above and beyond the parameters of his sources manifests in the strained repetition of a limited number of verbs that impart the sense of a forceful bludgeoning: Titus constantly "betiþ" (l. 539) the Jews who, in one passage alone, are "cloue" (l. 822), "hytte" (l. 825), "brayned" (l. 829), and "brosed" (l. 829) by their newly Christian enemies. It certainly seems that *The Siege of Jerusalem*, like *Cleanness*, is equating damnation with the destruction of the body's integrity, and engaging in a similarly negative, accusatory polemic.

Yet we must contextualize these descriptions of violence if we are to understand the tradition in which they appear. Violence in these stories relates directly to the metaphor of Christ the Physician, the vantage point from which the entire narrative strand must be understood. The poet figures violence against Jews as the logical conclusion of the spiritual sickness they incur by their betrayal of Christ. This refusal is seen as a disease, and the effects of violence, its symptoms. Yet it is not the scenes of violence that provide the poem with its symmetry and structure but those of healing. The converted Romans are the beneficiaries of an overdetermined wholeness, a salvationary emphasis that depends for its didactic force upon the contrasting example of the Jews. Indeed, there is little to distinguish the Romans from the Jews before the former convert to Christianity. The conditions afflicting Titus and Vespasian may be regarded as divine punishment for disbelief, just as chroniclers frequently depicted Vespasian's campaign against Jerusalem as a tool of God's vengeance against the disbelieving Jews.[112] The most important body in this poem does not belong to a Jewish subject of vengeance, or to a Roman recipient of grace, but to the suffering of Jesus Christ. Christ's body opens the poem because it is the ideal template of our own. This fragmented yet ultimately resurrected body that "al on rede blode ran" (l. 12) conditions our responses to the others in the poem. All that follows is part of a single, extended exemplar concerning the historical siege of Jerusalem, an episode often invoked in penitential contexts.[113] The focus of this poem is its exhortation to Christian faith, to sustained observance and adherence to Christ the Physician, not the violence against the Jews themselves.

This self-reflective motif is supported by the poem's manuscript contexts. The poem was often grouped with collections of chivalric and crusading romances, not surprising given its heroic flourishes and realistic descriptions of siege technology. It is for this reason that some scholars classify *The Siege of Jerusalem* as romance. Yet this poem was also often contained with religious texts, specifically the sort of *temporale* literature that generally employs the same dichotomizing strategy of representing saved and sinful bodies as, respectively, whole and fragmented. One such manuscript, British Library MS Additional 31042, contains both *The Siege of Jerusalem* and *The Northern Passion*. Bonnie Millar points out that these two texts are associated because, of the twenty-six items in the codex, they alone boast illustrations.[114] *The Northern Passion* is one of several fourteenth-century Middle English poems connecting the spectacle of Christ's Passion to the necessity of auricular confession. Not merely a means of provoking sympathy for Christ and indignation at his death, literary depictions of the Passion also served a practical purpose: to draw people to confession. For though Christ's wounded body was certainly a source of crude anti-Jewish sentiment, it was also, through the very fact of its renewal, the proof of confession's efficacy. In this poem, Christ warns the apostles of His impending Passion, stressing that although his bodily integrity will be brutally compromised in the crucifixion, "hale and sownde ȝe sall me se / In þe land of galyle."[115] A related poem, *A Stanzaic Life of Christ*, explicitly links the image of the Passion with the sacrament of confession: "hit mynnes on Cristes passioun / to excite monnes wille tho / to penaunce and contricion."[116] The extreme violence with which Christ's Passion is rendered in such works is therefore not a symptom of unrestrained bitterness against Jews, but it is a strategic device through which the mechanism of salvation can be precisely communicated. The seductive promise of wholeness that inheres in Christ's covenant with humanity depends for its force upon the corresponding image of the fragmented, damned body.

This dichotomy between wholeness and fragmentation finds powerful expression in another manuscript that combines *The Siege of Jerusalem* with more straightforwardly religious material. Huntington Library MS HM 128, a "predominantly religious collection," groups *The Siege of Jerusalem* with the immensely popular *The Pricke of Conscience*,[117] a poem that repeatedly states that the degree of bodily integrity one enjoys in the afterlife depends entirely on the quality of religious adherence he or she exhibits while alive. To quote one representative passage,

> And if any lym wanted, þat shuld falle
> Til þe body, or any war over smalle,
> Thurgh þe defaut here of kynd God þan wille
> Alle þe defautes of þe lyms fulfille,
> And þus sal he do namely to al þa
> þat sal be save and til blis ga.
>   (ll. 5008–5113)

In contrast to these saved bodies, sinners "sal alle unsemely be, / And foul, and ugly, opon to se" (ll. 5023–24). The characters in *The Siege of Jerusalem*, at various stages in their development, fall into one or the other of these two categories. Their decisions are reflected in their bodies, which betray their receipt or refusal of Christ the Physician's healing aid. In this sense, Malcolm Hebron's reading of the poem—that the sickness of Vespasian is thematically "a private recovery as well as a larger, more spiritual healing process"—registers only half the equation.[118] The healing of the Romans, and, by implication, of humanity in the Christian era, depends for its metaphorical force upon the corresponding descent of the Jews into a state of sickness. The Jews represent the unsaved state in which Vespasian and Titus would have remained had they not converted. As Ralph Hanna argues, the poem is not narrowly polemical, but "imagines a wider target, an unreconstructed paganism that includes both Roman and Jew."[119] Yet in perceiving both Romans and Jews as collectively a "target," Hanna understates the salvific message that underpins the action of the poem, which the poet realizes through the image of the thoroughly redemptive, healing surgeon.

It is not surprising that *The Siege of Jerusalem* would contain so much medical detail. This poem's subject matter turns, from its apocryphal beginnings, upon the overtly medical concept of *Christus Medicus*. To illustrate this point, we need look no further than the *Evangelium Nichodemi*, the poem's apocryphal source for the Jews' betrayal of Jesus. In the *Evangelium*, the original impetus for the betrayal of Christ is specifically medical: Jesus heals on the Sabbath. The Jews complain to Pontius Pilate that despite their injunction to the contrary, "this man of his Evil acts has cured on the sabbath, the lame and the deaf, the crippled and the paralytics, and the blind and the lepers and those possessed."[120] Pilate doubts the logic of condemning a man for performing good deeds, but the Jews demand justice and assure Pilate that "His blood be upon us and upon our children."[121] The holiness of Christ's healing is further illustrated by Satan's lament that those whom he "made blind, lame, cripples, lepers and mad, He cured with a word."[122] The Jews thus become, in their condemnation of Christ, aligned with Satan, setting the stage for the dichotomy between Christian and Jew, saved and unsaved, which informs all subsequent versions of the Matter of Jerusalem.

In all the versions of the story, Vespasian's disease is described as not only extremely unpleasant but also incurable. This emphasis upon the incurability of Vespasian has its origins in Eusebius's *Ecclesiastical History*, the source for this episode. In this work, Eusebius reproduces what he claims were originally letters exchanged between Jesus and a certain King Agbar, in which Agbar begs Christ, whom he has heard can "cleanse lepers," to cure his own suffering, which is "beyond human power to heal."[123] Shortly thereafter, a follower of Jesus heals Agbar, who swears passionately that he now has "such belief in him as to have wished to take force and destroy the Jews who crucified him."[124] Such a description suggests that leprosy is the specific culprit. This specificity is restated in the *Vindicta Salvatoris*, a frequent addendum to the *Evangelium*, in which Tiberius, assuming Agbar's role, "was ill with ulcers, very full of fever, which is the ninth kind of leprosy."[125] However, later accounts of this same story are often far more vague. In *The Siege of Jerusalem*, we are only told that Vespasian is afflicted with a "biker" (l. 32), inside which nests a horde of wasps. This condition is so horrible that "no leche vpon lyue" nor "grace growyng" could heal his "grym sores" (ll. 39–40). Yet the poet gives us no indication as to what causes these wounds. Jacobus de Voragine's version of the episode in his *Golden Legend* is similarly ambiguous; Vespasian has not only a wound full of wasps, but also a "botche ful of wormes."[126] Some versions, however, retain the specific medical context of leprosy, as does *The English Bible*, which explicitly refers to Vespasian as a "mezel."[127] Again, this specificity is played out more thoroughly in the fifteenth-century romance *Titus and Vespasian*, which has Vespasian in "meselrye soo depe" that he "sawe noon oþur þan to dye."[128] It would seem, then, that the medieval audience was accustomed to associating Vespasian's affliction with leprosy.

Significantly, religious writers often appropriate the disease of leprosy as a metaphor for damnation. One Middle English sermon, in discussing this "most wikkyd" of afflictions, describes the terrifying condition of the "vicius lepir of dedli synne," which can only be cured if one "shrife" and "be sori and repentaunt."[129] Not surprisingly, medieval moralists, concerned to promote virtuous behavior and frequent confession, often identified leprosy's cause as the commission of deadly sin, usually pride or lechery. The confessional manual *Of Shrifte and Penance*, for example, argues that "Lechurs vseth comune wymmen," and in the process "leze here soule," "dystryeth here body," and "leprus mesel ofte þey bycomyth."[130] The frequency with which such assertions occur in religious contexts often leads literary scholars to overstate the degree to which medieval society as a whole participated in this association between leprosy and sin. For example, Bryon Grigsby, whose recent monograph *Pestilence in Medieval and Early Modern Literature* provides important insights into the didactic value leprosy had for religious writers, argues that "these moral associations were literal," so that "when medieval people stated that envy caused leprosy, they meant that this sin literally caused leprosy."[131] While this was certainly true of clerical writers such as the author of *Of Shrifte and Penance*, it does not apply to "medieval people" universally. Indeed, the actual doctors charged with the grim yet essential task of examining patients for the disease did not tend to share this reductive approach to epidemiology. In an important yet often unheeded article, Luke Demaitre convincingly dismantles this nearly axiomatic convention of "inferring that medieval physicians sanctioned the moral overtones which indisputably dominated the treatment of leprosy in the literary, devotional, and popular sources."[132] According to Demaitre, medieval physicians recognized the erratic behavior of lepers not as the manifestation of those sins that lead to disease but rather of the undeniable shock of coping with both the onset of fatal illness and the social marginalization it entails.[133] Furthermore, the references in penitential writings to sores and blemishes have little in common with the far more precise and involved instructions for diagnosis provided by such authorities as Bernard Gordon and Guy de Chauliac.[134] Yet Grigsby is correct to identify the ubiquity of the association between leprosy and sin at the level of popular religion: writers and preachers so commonly insisted on the causal relationship between spiritual corruption and leprous wounds that this simplistic construction was to some degree internalized by the general population. In a society so saturated with the penitential rhetoric of fragmentation and redemption, such associations were perhaps inevitable. Indeed, as Caroline Bynum notes, the anxiety surrounding the leprous body was attributable to the fact that such bodies literally "fragmented and putrefied" and resembled "living death."[135] For the medievals, there could be no more potent reminder that the opposite of salvation, with its accompanying promise of wholeness, is the horrible fragmenting of the damned.

If we assume Vespasian's condition to be leprosy, then this puts into even sharper contrast the salvation of the Romans with the damnation of the Jews. The disease of leprosy was understood to be largely hereditary. Trevisa, for example, states that leprosy often "comeþ [of] fadir and modir, and so þis contagioun passiþ into þe childe as it were by lawe of heritage."[136] This disease, then, corresponds strongly to the sins of the Jews, which commentators often described as passed down through lineage. In *Titus and Vespasian*, a poem dealing with much of the same material as *The Siege of Jerusalem*, the fatal sin that Pilate commits in his betrayal of Christ taints not only himself but also the Jews and their bloodlines:

And ȝet smerte Pilate noght allone,
But þe Jewes everychone;
For þei bad his blood shulde falle
On hem and on her children alle.
　　　　　　(ll. 1583–86)

Such a description should not surprise anyone. The *Evangelium Nichodemi* argues that "the Jews through their envy have punished their descendants with a cruel condemnation."[137] Yet *Titus and Vespasian* goes on to place this generational schema within a specifically medical context, invoking the popular belief amongst medieval Christians that "a flour of blode" afflicts the Jews every Friday as a reminder of their sins, and this affliction will continue to torment the Jews until such time "as þei wil bileve" (ll. 1589, 1598). Such a formulation depends upon the view of Christ as Physician, and, indeed, the poet of *Titus and Vespasian* makes explicit his use of this pervasive trope by arguing that He assumed human form to "hele þe seke þat bilevede righte" (l. 1348). The Jews, who lack this vital faith, cut themselves off from receiving His ministrations, and they remain both physically and spiritually diseased. Their failure to accept His help is the cause of their continuing afflictions throughout all the versions of the Matter of Jerusalem. Conversely, the Romans, because they accept that which the Jews condemn, are endowed with symbolically exaggerated health throughout.

The Siege of Jerusalem establishes its context of health and illness from the very beginning. Vespasian, as we have seen, suffers from leprosy, a disease that medieval surgeons widely thought incurable by any earthly means. Guy de Chauliac warns surgeons from the outset that "it is noȝt alwaie in a leche to releue þe seke man," and posits lepers as the foremost example.[138] For his part, Titus's face is marred by a horrible "canker vnclene" (l. 30). The turning point for both characters comes when Titus encounters Nathan, a seafarer from Jerusalem whose boat has been swept ashore at Rome, and asks,

> What medecyn is most, þat þat may vseþ,
> Wheþer gommes, oþer graces, or any goode drenches,
> Oþer chauntementes, or charmes? y charge þe to say.
> (ll. 94–96)

Nathan informs the desperate Roman of Veronica's veil, claiming that there is no "[m]eselry ne meschef" that cannot be cured if the afflicted but "kneleþ doun to þat cloþ & on Crist leueþ" (ll. 166–67). Titus, instantly believing this story, and vowing to avenge his newfound Savior against the Jews who betrayed him, is immediately healed. Vespasian quickly hears of this miracle and desires a similar release. Pope Peter touches him lightly with the veil, saying a prayer three times (l. 250), and Vespasian, instantly cured of his illness, declares that he "mychel Crist loued" (l. 273). This healing, while miraculous, initiates an extended metaphor of surgery as divine salvation that persists throughout the poem. Veronica had long been associated with miraculous healing, and her claim to have obtained the impression directly from Christ's bloody face was authenticated by Pope Innocent III in the thirteenth century. As Eve Kuryluk has noted, the legend of Veronica derives from the New Testament account of the anonymous woman with the flux of blood, and it carries great symbolic force because it constitutes "a marvel of symmetry: the man whose cloth has stopped the woman's bleeding has his own flux of blood which she arrests with her cloth."[139] Yet this is also a story of contraries: the woman's corrupt menstrual blood meets its opposite in Christ's perfected blood, and the resulting healing anticipates Titus's cure by contraries in the latter half of the poem. More immediately, however, Veronica's veil suggests the medical charm, a treatment frequently used in surgical practice and itself based on the principle of contraries. Charms are ritualized incantations that purport to heal wounds by invoking the name of Christ, of Mary, or of one of the various saints. Most often, chants are performed in conjunction with an amulet or plate bearing an inscription of one of these holy names, and they are meant to transmit to that object the healing power of the subject of adjuration. Significantly, Veronica is one of the saints frequently called upon in such healing verbalizations. For example, in the *Rosa Medicinae* of John Gaddesden there is a charm that instructs the user to write the name "Veronica" on the sick person's forehead, and then to say, "we humbly implore you Lord Jesus Christ, who alone cures the sick, to lift the right hand of your power and holiness and restrict and stop the flow of blood of this person for whom we pour forth our prayers."[140] Vespasian's cure by means of the veil resembles the use of the surgical charm in several respects. For one, Peter repeats the healing action three times. As Carole Rawcliffe has suggested, the number three often inhered in the performance of charms because it invoked, at least implicitly, the added protection of the Trinity.[141] Second, Peter touches Vespasian with the veil, an action necessary to distinguish his ministrations from a simple prayer. The use of some mediating implement is a central feature of this type of remedy. An example is the "uncorrupted wounds of Christ" charm, which George Keiser surmises is the oldest surviving example of the genre in English.[142] This charm instructs the user to engrave onto a plate five crosses, one for each of Christ's wounds, then to say five paternosters. One example of this charm, contained in what appears to be a medieval practitioner's notebook, purports to be "medecyne verrey to warych manne wonde if he be not wounded to þe dede," and claims that just as Christ's wounds did not fester, hurt, or stink, so also the wounds of the recipient of this charm need not be subject to such conditions.[143] Christ's healing power is a component of God's grace, and, as such, was unavailable to Vespasian before his conversion. According to the confessional manual *Speculum Christiani*, the "body of Cryste es medecyn to seke men," through which we are made "more buxum to correpcion."[144] Through this implicit allusion to the medical charm, the poet places the very launch point of the narrative, Vespasian's miraculous conversion, in a demonstrably medical context.

Significantly, it is at this point in the narrative that the poet returns to the imagery of Christ's Passion. Newly healed, Titus and Vespasian travel with the Roman army to Jerusalem to confront the Jews. After failing several times to obtain a Jewish surrender, the Romans meet their enemy on the field. Before the battle begins, Vespasian addresses the Roman troops, while Caiaphas addresses the Jews; to motivate their men, they invoke the core motifs of their respective faiths. In what Elisa Narin van Court has aptly called "a striking textual moment of oppositions,"[145] Vespasian recounts the Passion of Christ, a visceral image par excellence, and his opposite number invokes the more abstract concept of "Moyses lawe" (l. 480). Together, these constitute the "two central tropes of these two religions."[146] Vespasian appeals to the newfound faith of his men with an account of the Passion that would be at home in any penitential document:

> Beholdeþ þe heþyng & þe harde woundes,
> þe betyng & þe byndyng, þat þe body hadde:
> Lat neuer þis lawles ledis lauȝ at his harmys,
> þat bouȝt vs fram bale with blod of his herte.
>   (ll. 493–96)

Narin van Court makes much of this passage, identifying in its rhetoric the exegetical commonplace that, in place of Jewish law, there is now the grace that the image of the Passion paradigmatically signifies. We will recall the Rule of St. Augustine, where it is stated that Christians are "no longer slaves under the law," but they are "a people living in freedom under grace." Here, Vespasian appears to be mocking the stubborn continuation of Old Testament justice into this new salvationary era.

This passage also serves to make explicit the eschatological quality that resides in the poem's *Christus Medicus* motif. If the New Testament is the story of a Physician who has come to heal the spiritually sick, then what of the Old? A sermon contemporary with *The Siege of Jerusalem* provides an engaging answer:

> Frendis, Crist dois þis as þe grett fecicions and leches don when þat þei com owte of a farre countrey: þei aspie where þat oþur leches haue fayled, and þeþur þei goy and ȝeuen here medecyns for to shewe here connynge. Ryght so Crist Ihesu, when all prophetis be þe lawe of Moyses fayles for to saue mans sowle, for þat was þe lawe of vengeaunce, þan com Crist, and with is preciouse blode he made man hole. And so by is noyse þat he made on þe Crosse to is Fadur of heuen on Good Fridaye, he ȝaue liff to mans soule as doþ þe lion to is qwelpe.[147]

This passage, despite its clear metaphorical character, depends on the recognizable image of the foreign doctor for its power. Many municipalities in medieval England had a system in place for the regulation of visiting practitioners. In York in the fourteenth century, at least two of the names available from the meager records relating to medical practice were of foreign origin.[148] Indeed, this passage seems an inversion of the typically negative reaction of barber-surgeon guilds to such perceived encroachment, for example that of the barbers of London in an ordinance of 1375:

> [T]he good folk Barbers of the said city show that from day to day there come from Uppelande, Men, Barbers, little skilled in their craft, into the said city, and take houses and intermeddle with barbery, surgery, and with the cure of other sicknesses, whereas they know not how to do such things nor ever were qualified in that carft to the great damage and cheating of the people and to the great scandal of all the honest barbers of the said city.[149]

The frequency with which the transition from the Old to the New Testament was conveyed in the context of healing would have made Vespasian's speech resonate with medical meaning, especially given the earlier reference to medicinal charms. Vespasian, after all, has been healed because of Nathan, a foreigner whose very birthplace, Jerusalem, associates him with miraculous cures. For Vespasian, the notion of Christ the Physician is no mere rhetoric to spur on his men, for Vespasian himself has direct experience of Christ's healing, of "bale with blod of his herte."

Although the second set of healings is surgical rather than divine, Christ's wounded body as invoked by Vespasian tidily conflates these miraculous and secular manifestations of grace. After an initial skirmish in which the Romans emerge victorious, the Jews barricade themselves in the city. A group of them, however, tunnel under the walls at an unexpected location and ambush the Romans; a second battle ensues. In this conflict, Vespasian receives a wound to the foot that the poet describes as "wonder-lich sore" (l. 811). The poet had a choice of two very different accounts to use for this wounding. In *The Jewish Wars* by Josephus, a Jewish chronicler who left his countrymen to align himself with the Romans,[150] Vespasian's wound is not at all serious. Because of the long range the arrow had to travel, the "wound was slight," and the initial concern of the troops was soon replaced by their desire to "avenge their commander."[151] In the fourteenth-century *Polychronicon* by Ranulphus Higden, however, Vespasian fares much worse. As Trevisa translates it, he is "sore wounded in the hele," and effectively removed from the fighting.[152] The poet's choice of the latter version, in which the wound is far graver, creates the context in which medical personnel may be called in. Although Josephus does mention physicians in his *Antiquities*, and though they were present at the historical siege, there is no evidence for actual medical treatment at the battles themselves.[153] Bonnie Millar has argued that the poet magnifies the seriousness of Vespasian's injury so that the Jewish "stratagems are rendered more prominent, highlighting the devious tricks of the Jews."[154] This is in keeping with the conventional interpretation that the poem is ultimately concerned with the folly of the Judaic people. Yet the addition of surgical treatment to the scene of Vespasian's wounding is entirely original, and is meant to emphasize not the evil of the Jews, but rather the virtue of the Christians, whose access to grace is the direct result of their conversion.

This element of grace inheres in the very terms of the poet's description of the surgery on the Romans. Immediately following Vespasian's injury, the Romans run roughshod over their opponents in a passage that boasts the poem's most concentrated description of violence (ll. 821–32). The various fragmentations inflicted here, including the tearing of stomachs, breaking of skulls, and decapitations, are meant to contrast with the subsequent depiction of surgical treatment, which is enclosing rather than fragmenting. While the Jews are incurable, the Romans are vigorously tended to:

> Waspasian stynteþ of þe stour, steweþ his burnes,
> þat wer for-beten & bled vnder bryȝt yren;
> Tyen to her tentis myd tene þat þey hadde,
> Al wery of þat werk & wounded ful sore.
> Helmes & hamberkes hadden of sone,
> Leches by torche-liȝt loken her hurtes,
> Waschen woundes with wyn & with wolle stoppen,
> With oyle & orisoun ordeyned in charme.
>
> (ll. 841–48)

We will recall that while still a pagan, there was no "leche vpon lyue" to whom Vespasian could turn. It is when Nathan tells Titus of Jesus, who "leched at enys" (l. 122), that they become subjects of grace. Now, this grace is again realized in the ministrations of the "leches" who treat Vespasian and the other wounded. An academic surgeon like Guy de Chauliac would disdain this simple battlefield surgery, along with "alle knyghtes of Saxoun and of men folowynge batailles, the whiche procuren or helen alle woundes with coniurisouns and drynkes and with oyle and wolle and a cole leef, foundynge ham therfore vppon that, that God putte his vertu in herbes, wordes and stones."[155] According to Guy de Chauliac, only women and fools make worse surgeons than knightly amateurs. Indeed, this passage echoes Guy's description to a remarkable degree: "oyle," "wolle," and "charme" are all mentioned as techniques used to heal the Romans. Yet the professionalism of these practitioners is very much in evidence. The poet is careful to mention that the surgeons "loken her hurtes" before acting, an emphasis upon diagnosis in keeping with the advice of the major surgical authorities. As William of Saliceto cautions, the failure to properly view the wound constitutes an "ignoraunce of ser-chynge"; if as a result the wrong treatment is applied, there can be severe consequences: "þe schapp and maner of þe membres shul be distroyed."[156] Surgical treatment can kill as easily as heal, a range of possibilities that further serves to conflate successful surgery with the grace of God. Furthermore, as we have seen, this practice of viewing the wound to its bottom often served as a metaphor for full confession, an association that strengthens the redemptive emphasis of the poem as a whole. De Chauliac would also have objected to the simplicity of this treatment: that the wounds are "stoppen" with wool and left to heal. This immediate stopping of wounds became the dominant practice in military surgery, even as such seemingly cursory measures were hotly debated in scholastic circles for their opposition to the prevailing medical theory that wounds should be healed by *secondary intention* alone.[157] That is, wounds were thought to heal best if kept open and their dressings changed frequently, so that corrupt humors could escape the orifice. Only when the surgeon could see *laudable pus* running from the wound was it healed. Such pus was thought to be formed by an influx of vital heat, whose presence signified that the wound was no longer blocked by corrupt humoral matter, but could safely be allowed to close. In times of war, however, surgeons discovered—no doubt through sheer repetition—the utility of immediate closure and infrequent dressing. Henri de Mondeville was a major proponent of this passive techniques, but he was outnumbered by those authorities who resented this challenge to medical orthodoxy.[158] Yet this stopping of wounds has a deeper import. The application of bandages to an abrasion was a frequent metaphor in this period for the remedying of spiritual faults. The fourteenth-century Henry, duke of Lancaster, provides an extended example of this popular metaphor in his *Livres des seyntez medicines*, in which the penitent narrator prays to Jesus for "white cloths to wrap around myself, so that I do not lose the virtue of the good poultices and the holy ointments placed on my sores to heal them."[159] Indeed, in their descriptions of medicated dressings, or *plasters*, collectors of medical recipes would often blur the distinction between the metaphorical and the literal. One fourteenth-century recipe book contains a plaster called "godisgrace." Of all plasters, "he ys most helyng and most closiþ and hasterloker makeþ goud flesche wex," and "suffreþ no ded flesche ne no corrupcion of wounde."[160] This surgical application, in other words, performs the same cure as the medical charm and appeals to the same source of healing power—that is, God's mercy.

The intentional linking of Vespasian's two healings, the miraculous and the surgical, is perhaps best seen in the poet's transposition of the medical charm from one context to the other. Indeed, it is the first of de Chauliac's objections—the use of "coniurisouns"—that most links this surgical scene to the miraculous healings that open the poem. There is no better evidence that one cannot determine the nature of medieval medical practice through learned treatises alone than the wildly differing attitudes in the period toward medical charms. Guy de Chauliac objects strenuously to this type of remedy, and openly ridicules Gilbertus Anglicus for providing so many examples.[161] Nor was this prejudice restricted to medical authorities. In 1382, a London man was tried and found guilty for fraud after having sold a woman a written charm invoking the body and blood of Christ.[162] Many of the more sophisticated members of English society seemed to have little time for such folk-oriented remedies—in this, Geoffrey Chaucer is no exception. In the "General Prologue" to the *Canterbury Tales*, Chaucer endows his Physician with a thorough inventory of medical knowledge; he knows both "phisik and surgerie," including humoral pathology and diagnosis, astronomy, regimen, and pharmacy.[163] Yet nowhere does he mention charms, despite the fact that several authorities named in the list of books the physician has read advocate their use.[164] As the *Canterbury Tales* proceed, they reveal Chaucer as rather antagonistic toward charms and their users. The cuckolded carpenter of *The Miller's Tale* attempts to wake Nicholas from his feigned trance through a "nyght-spel," which invokes "Jheus Crist and Seinte Benedight."[165] In this case, those who believe in charms are made to look foolish and naïve, like the carpenter himself. Chaucer's Parson, on a more serious note, takes aim at "thilke horrible sweryng of adjuracioun and conjuracioun," and insists that if charms "for woundes" have any effect, "it may be paraventure that God siffreth it, for folk sholden yeve the moore feith and reverence to his name."[166] For the Parson, then, charms do not represent the visible expression of the grace of God, but rather a naïve and impious use of the language, images, and tropes of the Christian religion. It is likely that de Chauliac, as a cleric in lesser orders,[167] objected to such supernatural remedies because he viewed them from the Parson's clerical perspective, and saw them as appropriating, on a populist level, a salutary agenda thought to be the exclusive province of the Church alone.

Despite these objections, for many practitioners charms were not only acceptable but also a vital part of their medical repertoire. John Gaddesden, as we have seen, incorporated them into his *Rosa Medicinae*, and included one invoking Veronica. The Oxford-educated Gaddesden, the only major medical writer to emerge from an English university, addressed his book to surgeons and physicians alike, obviously intending both to make use of its material.[168] Another compendium, that of Gilbertus Anglicus, boasts of charms that staunch bleeding by invoking the wounds of Christ.[169] Both books were prominent in Austin libraries and could well have been known to the poet.[170] Although the survival of these remedies in written form does not mean they were actually used, the case of the fifteenth-century English practitioner Thomas Fayreford does indicate that charms were applied as part of standard medical practice. As Peter Jones has demonstrated, Fayreford, who left behind a commonplace book, "placed significant reliance on charms" and employed them against a variety of ailments.[171] Because both Fayreford and Gaddesden attended Oxford, their use of charms cannot be dismissed as characteristic of only uneducated or provincial physicians. Surgeons also included charms in their repertoires. Theodoric states as part of his instructions for a medicine "for patients suffering from wounds" that the surgeon should sprinkle the active ingredient onto the syrup base three times "in the shape of a cross," adding for good measure an accompanying prayer of the sort typical of other medical charms.[172] By invoking such charms in his description of the Roman surgery, the poet ensures that this episode and the earlier depictions of God's healing grace are understood as two sides of a single, salutary coin. Furthermore, the poet retains an emphasis upon surgery throughout as the medium through which God's grace works to render Vespasian and his fellow Romans indestructible.

There is a similar continuity between the two healings of Titus. Again, we are meant to view surgery as an extension of God's grace, and its healing effects as a metaphor for the rewards of salvation. Titus is so overjoyed at Vespasian's assumption of the imperial throne that he suffers sudden paralysis. When he is told of his father's good fortune, "in his synwys soudeynly a syknesse is fallen" (l. 1024). This condition afflicts Titus with cramps in all of his joints, causing him to become "croked aȝens kynde," and "as a crepel" (l. 1029). Such paralysis is by no means an invention on the part of the poet. Scholastic medical theory often attested to the idea that an influx of emotion can upset an individual's delicate humoral balance through the loss of his body's vital heat. For example, the twelfth-century Jewish philosopher and medical authority Moses Maimonides, in his influential *Regimen of Health*, explains that

> passions of the psyche produce changes in the body, that are great, evident, and manifest to all. As evidence thereof, you can see a man of robust build, ringing voice, and glowing face, when there reaches him, unexpectedly, news that afflicts him greatly. You will observe, that all of a sudden his color dims, the brightness of his face departs, he loses stature, his voice becomes hoarse, and even if he strives to raise his voice he cannot, his strength diminishes and often he trembles from the magnitude of the weakness, his pulse diminishes, his eyes sink, his eyelids become too heavy to move, the surface of his body cools, and his appetite subsides. The cause of all these signs is a recall of the natural heat and the blood into the interior of the body. . .On this account the physicians have directed that concern and care should always be given to the movements of the psyche; these should be kept in balance in the state of health as well as in disease, and no other regimen should be given precedence in any wise.[173]

Maimonides's prescription for such a condition—that the patient should be treated with regard to "the movements of the psyche"—forms the basis of the cure that Titus eventually receives. His company, concerned with this sudden deterioration in their leader's health, searches the city in vain for any physician who has survived the siege. Finally, his men enlist Josephus, "þat surgyan was noble" (l. 1035). Josephus prescribes treatment by contraries, which, in this case, amounts to the provocation in Titus of feelings of hate and distress, rather than of joy.[174] By placing at the dinner table a man whom Titus virulently despises, Josephus causes Titus to experience a "hote yre" whose corresponding physical effects are to restore vital heat and repair his shrunken veins and sinews (ll. 1046–50).

Titus, as we have seen, has already suffered from, and been healed of, a cancerous growth. In this second instance, Titus is afflicted with, and is cured of, a sickness that renders him "croked aȝens kynde." These two conditions correspond precisely to Nathan's descripiton of Christ's healing powers, those very words through which Titus was first cured of cancer and brought to conversion. Jesus, according to Nathan, cures all those who are "[c]roked & cancred" (l. 125). Titus, cured now of both these conditions, personifies the spiritual and physical healing that is the reward of Christianity. In this remarkably economical fashion, the poet illustrates for the reader the necessity of conforming to Christ through an earthly healing that he conveys to his audience with all the force of parable. Indeed, the exemplary collection *An Alphabet of Tales* would invoke this same episode as an example of the virtue of forgiveness.[175] Titus forgives both the man he hates and also Josephus, who, because a Jew, was previously his enemy. This secular healing lends itself particularly well to such a moral lesson precisely because it employs the principle of contraries. The medieval medical truism that a particular humoral superfluity is best negated through the application of its opposite had long been marshaled in the service of moral exposition.[176] St. Augustine, for instance, posits a "Christian medicine" in which the example of Christ negates our vices with virtues, just like a physician who "applies certain opposites, as cold to hot, wet to dry."[177] Surgeons had long observed this principle in their own treatments. William of Saliceto, for one, informs his readers that "if eny mater holden inne þe disposicion, þe remouynge of þe same schal be cause of distroyinge of þilke disposicion, and so aftirward þe manere of þis curacion is clepid þe contrarius."[178] *A Stanzaic Life of Christ*, written in Chester and based on the same sources as *The Siege of Jerusalem*,[179] describes Christ's negation of the sins of Adam with reference to this surgical commonplace:

> And vset ys most communely
> contrarius medicyn forto dight
> in fisik and in surgery,
> who-ser wol hele a sore oright.
> > (ll. 6265–6268)

The poet seems to have been influenced by such popular metaphors. In declaring Josephus a "surgyan," *The Siege of Jerusalem* departs not only from *The Golden Legend*, its apparent source for this episode, but also from any tradition of which I am aware. Indeed, William Caxton's *Game of Chess*, a translation of Jacobus de Cessolis's *Liber de ludo scaccorum*, (Book on the Game of Chess) recounts this same episode, but instead refers to Josephus as "a right wyse phisicien."[180] The surgeon applies contraries not only in his use of plasters, drugs, and cauteries, but also in his recitation of charms—after all, charms counter the dissolution of our fallen flesh through the invocation of Christ's own, indissoluble body. Indeed, Titus credits Christ with this restoration of his health when he "þonkeþ God of his grace & þe goode leche / Of alle" (ll. 1051–52). In this poem, then, it is not *Christus Medicus* who provides for our continuing health and potential for both bodily and spiritual salvation, but, remarkably, *Christus chirurgicus* [Christ the Surgeon].

The release of these two Christian converts from disease and injury suggests the benefits of sustained Christian observance in general. Indeed, the poet implements this broad lesson in the necessity of faith by extending the imperviousness of his two main characters to the Roman army as a whole. Despite the fact that the Jewish defenders are described as formidable—as "Fresche vnfonded folke" that "grete defence made" (ll. 618)—the Romans are, throughout their battles with the Jews, strangely unharmed. After the first, pivotal battle, they are just "as þey fram Rome come" (l. 605). Even after numerous, deadly skirmishes, the Romans remain "frescher to fiȝt þan at þe furst tyme" (l. 858). The repetition throughout of the word "clene" alerts us to the connection in the poem between spiritual purity and physical intactness. Just as the converted Titus "clenly was heled" of his cancer, so too is the unharmed army of Rome described as the "knyȝthode clene þat for Crist werred" (l. 856). Titus, before his "clene" healing, exists in a state of spiritual *un*cleanness, a state realized physically by his "canker vnclene" (l. 30). As in *Cleanness*, then, "clene" has the connotation not only of spiritual health but of bodily health as well. This twofold designation of health helps to separate not only the virtuously intact Romans from the horribly wounded Jews, but also the post-conversion Romans from their previous, spiritually unhealthy selves. The spiritual condition of the Jews is confirmed in the brutal wounds that they receive from the Romans.

In contrast to the intact Romans, the Jews are opened with such stultifying frequency that the effect is jarringly dichotomous. The application of plasters and other coverings to the wounded body amounts to a virtuous enclosure, and therefore contrasts with the image of the sinfully perforated body. Medically, this distinction between the irrevocable wounds of the Jews and the treatable ones of the Romans has much to do with the differentiations surgeons made between various sorts of wounds in their writings. Wounds were broadly divided into two categories, the *simple* and the *compound*. A simple wound is one in which the sinews have not been breached. Compound wounds, on the other hand, are far direr. Among the sorts of accidents that can cause simple wounds, Lanfranco lists those that, like Vespasian's dart wound, arise from projectiles, such as "spere or arowe, or wiþ ony oþir þing semblablele to hem."[181] For this sort of injury, Lanfranco recommends only that the surgeon "closiþ þe wounde togideris," because, in such straightforward cases, "þer nediþ noon oþer cure."[182] Simple wounds can be cured so easily because of the body's natural ability to create blood, which, in turn, contains the vital heat necessary for the regeneration of lost flesh. As Lanfranco explains, "blood is engendrid al day in us, & þe blood is þe mater of þe fleisch."[183] The Jews, of course, are not so lucky. Their blood consistently empties from their bodies, coloring the battlefield with implausible rivers of gore. The blood of the Jews "goutes fram gold wede as goteres" (l. 560), and "fomed hem fro in þe flasches aboute" (l. 571). These wounds the Jews receive, unlike the simple wounds of the Romans, result not in that which is merely pierced or lacerated, but, as Lanfranco puts it, in "þat, þat is departid."[184] In these cases, the possibility of healing is utterly foreclosed, since, when "membris of office ben kutt of, þei moun neuere be restorid."[185] There can be no regeneration of flesh, and therefore no healing, for these enemies of the Romans. Resurrection, the reward of all observant Christians, is denied the Jews, and this exemption is inscribed brutally onto their bodies. Like lepers, these irreparably wounded Jews function as living reminders of the necessity of receiving and maintaining God's grace, an imagistic strategy in keeping with the pragmatic "doctrine of tolerance" that, as Narin Van Court has demonstrated, animates the poem as a whole.

Nowhere in the poem is this contrast between intact Romans and wounded Jews more apparent than in its deliberate juxtaposition of two dichotomous images: the arming of Vespasian and the flaying of Caiaphas. On the third day of the siege the poet presents us with a conventional arming scene, moving from "þe fote to þe fourche" (l. 742) with all the opulence of romance. We see Vespasian enclose himself in a breastplate of "gray steel & of golde riche," a "grete girdel," and a "gold hewen helme," topped by a crown "ful of riche stones" (ll. 745–58). The effect is to lend Vespasian an appearance of indestructibility that accords with his status as a subject of grace and that matches the wealth and power with which one who believes in Christ is figuratively endowed.[186] More importantly, however, this image also stands as the symbolic counterpoint to the passage that immediately precedes it, which depicts the brutal punishing of Caiaphas and the Jewish commanders. These Jews are sentenced by the Romans to be "quyk flayn," then anointed with honey to encourage clawed, hungry animals to further "renten þe rawe flesche vpon rede peces" (ll. 694, 702). The defenses of Vespasian's armor are therefore contrasted with the body of Caiaphas, which, in its flayed state, is no longer covered by the skin that, according to Trevisa, "defendiþ al þe inner parties."[187] Medically, the skin was thought vulnerable to deterioration through the body's expulsion of corrupt humoral matter. These expelled humors, because pushed out through the pores, cause severe surface conditions, such as "stripinge and huldinge, and with mony sore greues."[188] The flaying of the Jews is a symptom of their original, fatal disorder, incurred in their betrayal of Christ. Just as Vespasian's overdetermined health extends to the entire Roman army as a symbol of the benefits of grace, so too does its imagistic opposite, the brutal flaying of Caiaphas, suggest the collective damnation of the unconverted Jews.

This vulnerability of the Jews finds further figurative expression through their frequent comparison to architectural structures. Metaphorically, the incredulous Jews are subjects of a faith founded on unfinished, and therefore brittle, foundations. The following example conflates their bodies with the fallible structures they inhabit, implicitly commenting on their foreclosure of eternal wholeness in the afterlife:

> Burnes wer brayned & brosed to deþ,
> Wymmen wide open walte vnder stones,
> Frosletes fro þe ferst to þe flor þrylled,
> & many toret doun tilte þe temple a-boute.
> (ll. 829–32)

The Jews are frequently conflated in this manner with the city they defend. These two separate exertions of force, against buildings and against bodies, are described almost identically, suggesting that we are meant to associate each with the other. One Jew's "herte *brestyþ*" [bursteth] from famine because of the long duration of the Roman offensive (l. 1082), while Caiaphas, the Jewish leader, is bound so tightly that his "blode out *barst*" (l. 586). The poet applies this same language he uses to describe the assault on the bodies of the Jews to the city itself. In their attack on the city walls, the Romans "*[b]rosten* þe britages & þe brode toures" (l. 658), while themselves suffering "noȝt a ryng *brosten*" (l. 606). Other such links between bodies and buildings occur throughout the poem. Titus "*betiþ* on harde" the bodies of the Jews (l. 539), just as his victorious army "doun *betyn* & brent into blake erþe" (l. 1288) the undefended city walls. Similarly, Titus, while again in combat with the Jews, "þe helm & þe hed *hewen* at-tonys" (l. 1123), just as the Romans, in breaching the walls, "*Hewen* þrow hard ston" (l. 1279). This deliberate comparison of the Jews to stones is not unique. Indeed, Jacobus de Voragine adopts this very metaphor to express the relationship of the Jews to the Son of God whom they have betrayed: "O ye Jewes ye be stones but ye smyte a better stone, wherof resowneth the sowne of pyte & boylleth the oyle of charyte."[189] Without salvation, the body is no more impervious to tribulation than anything else in the transient, fallen world.

This comparison of the Jews to architectural structures is very much in keeping with the tradition of medieval anatomical description, which consistently images the body as an architectural structure. The medieval understanding of the body is, of course, very different from our own. The workings of the body were tied inextricably to the surrounding cosmos, subject to a uniformity of self and space that contradicts thoroughly the firm ontological divisions that characterize our own, post-Cartesian conceptions of the relationship between the individual and the universe. The divine order that pervaded, structured, and ruled over the natural world also governed the internal workings of the body. It is not surprising, then, to find the internal described with recourse to external structures. Trevisa does so throughout his extensive anatomical description, referring to the stomach as the "dore" of the womb, the legs as "pileres," and the bones as the "foundement" supporting the "byldyng of al þe body."[190] Frequently, these architectural comparisons assume a distinctly martial character. Hence, according to Isidore of Seville, the eyelids are "roofs" defending the eyes, "fortified by a rampart of hairs, so that anything striking even against the open eyes will be repelled."[191] This motif of defensive enclosure pervades all medieval anatomical writings. The head is said to defend the brain, the back to defend the organs, and so on. According to Trevisa, the back is hard "as it were a stone," necessary for the "defens and helynge of þe inner parties."[192] This conception of the body as an edifice can be seen to inform Vespasian's promise to ensure "þat neuer ston in þat stede stond vpon oþer" (l. 978), and to render the violent sentiment of this promise both economical and encompassing. If we accept as commonplace, for example, Trevisa's analogy that "þe forhede is þe tour and þe defens" of the brain (l. 188), then the seemingly distinct images of the Jews being "brayned" (l. 829) and their "brode toures" (l. 658) destroyed become disturbingly twinned. In both cases, violence takes the form of the fragmenting of the previously intact structure, the very fate of the damned in the afterlife.

This association finds further expression in the writings of Vitruvius, the second-century architect who remained, throughout the Middle Ages, the towering authority for that art's practitioners. Vitruvius influentially held up the body as the standard of proportion to which all buildings should aspire. This is especially true of his discussion of symmetry:

> Symmetry is a proper agreement between the members of the work itself, and relation between the different parts and the whole general scheme, in

accordance with a certain part selected as standard. This is the human body there is a kind of symmetrical harmony between forearm, foot, palm, finger, and other small parts; and so it is with perfect buildings.[193]

This body-as-architecture metaphor would influence all subsequent discourses on aesthetics throughout the Middle Ages, including those of Thomas Aquinas and Vincent de Beauvais.[194] Tellingly, this divinely ordained symmetry is the very aspect of the body that the surgeon is charged with protecting. According to Lanfranco, two of the surgeon's duties are the "remeuynge of þat, þat is to myche," such as growths and swellings, and "bringyng to her placis ioyntis þat ben oute."[195] The surgeon, in other words, must maintain the very symmetry that governs Vitruvius's principles of architecture. As we have seen, medieval classifications of knowledge often conflated medicine with architecture, since both must combine a profound a priori knowledge with mechanical dexterity. Just as the surgeon, according to Lanfranco, must ensure the removal of any "superfluyte" from the body, so too does Vitruvius insist that in the construction of buildings "superfluity is useless."[196] It is not surprising, given the cross-fertilization of these two discourses, that Vitruvius demands of the architect "knowledge of the study of medicine."[197] Indeed, this connection persists well into the Middle Ages. The lodge book of the twelfth-century architect Villard de Honecourt contains an array of human forms amongst its drawings, and it even boasts a remedy for healing wounds.[198] Since Villard's is the only surviving example, there is no reason to assume that its contents are not characteristic of other, lost examples. While many members of medieval professions, including bookkeepers and accountants, collected remedies in the course of their daily business, the aforementioned centrality of the body and medicine to writings on architecture renders Villard de Honecourt's example particularly resonant. Medieval architecture regarded the integrity of the body as very much related to that of buildings, and the craft of the architect to that of the surgeon.

If the integrity of a building suggests the intact and healthy body, then the besieged Jewish city of *The Siege of Jerusalem*, pierced and punctured as it is, must stand as that body's unhealthy opposite. This *non*integrity would have been especially resonant to a society that associated the spectacle of healing miracles with completed, or repaired, buildings. In a letter of 1145, Hugh d'Amiens, the archbishop of Rouen, recounts with wonder the healings that occurred amongst the volunteers helping to repair a Church at Chartres. According to d'Amiens, "they commenced in humility to draw carts and beams for the construction of the church," during which time "very many miracles took place in our churches, and the sick who had come with them were made whole."[199] According to d'Amiens, the sick were laid upon the same wagons as the stones used in the repairs, and these folk, "vexed with divers diseases, arise whole from the wagons on which they had been laid."[200] As the holes in the church were repaired, so, too, were the infirmities, and presumably the wounds, of the sick. There is, then, a direct correlation between the sanctity of stones and of bodies. The materiality of each is transformed through the grace of Christ; the metaphorical collapses into the literal. As William Durand, for a time the bishop of Mende, argues in his *Rationale divinorum officiorum*, "as the material church is constructed from the joining together of various stones, so is the Spiritual Church by that of various men."[201] For the Jews of *The Siege of Jerusalem*, the possibility of such virtuous intactness, either on the level of the body or of the buildings that represent it, is perilously foreclosed. The state of wandering the Jews incur through their continued disbelief stands in stark opposition to Christian salutary aesthetics, which frequently depict salvation as a state of walled enclosure. Indeed, religious writers often depicted heaven as just such a walled city, an enclosed community of the faithful, a concept so ingrained in medieval Christian thought that it was conventionally the last sentiment imparted to the dying. One Latin service book of the fifteenth century contains the following English fragment, which outlines "how mene þat bene in hele sulde visite sike men":

> My dere sone or douȝtere in god, hyt semith þat þou hyest þe faste in þe wey
> fro þis life to godward, þere þou schalt cee al þy forme-fadris, apostelis,
> martiris, confessouris and uirgynis, & all men and wommen þat ben saued;
> and fore gladnes of suche felauschip be þou of good confort in god, þynke
> how þou muste after þis lyfe leye a stone in þe wall of þe cite of heuene,
> sclely with outen noise or strife, and þerfore, or þou wende out of þis world,
> þou polissch þi stoon and make it redi, ȝif þou wolt not þere be lettid.[202]

We see, then, that salvation was often equated with entrance into a city, a spatial metaphor that rendered accessible the important spiritual concept of "dying well" by comparing that ethereal journey to the common experience of passing through municipal boundaries. If indeed an Austin Canon, our poet may well have encountered the following words from a fellow canon living at Barnwell Priory: "Even as a lofty tower surrounded on all sides by walls makes the soldiers who garrison it safe, fearless, and impregnable, so the Rule of blessed Augustine, fortified on all sides by observances in accordance with it, makes its soldiers—that is, the regular canons— undismayed at the attacks of the devil, safe and invincible."[203] The various, oppositional images of enclosures and openings that occur throughout *The Siege of Jerusalem* relate to this integral dichotomy between the saved and the damned. More importantly, however, they serve to promote a correspondingly secure Christian identity. To return to Fisher and Cleveland, "the body is experienced as an approximate replica of some of the basic internalized systems" that constitute the individual's sense of self.[204] If *Cleanness* attacks this selfhood through a sustained focus on the wounded, sinful body, then *The Siege of Jerusalem* takes the opposite approach, confirming for the faithful the corporeal and spiritual benefits of continued adherence to Christ. Its vehicle for doing so is the ambivalent figure of the surgeon, who could stand not only for the horrible de-partitioning of the damned—their pain, terror, and despair at the irrevocable loss of God—but also for the protection and joy of the saved: in other words, for the benefits of salvation itself.

Conclusion

Beginning with Plato, pagan philosophers vaunted the mechanical arts as both the province of, and path back to, the Divine Mind. With the arrival of St. Augustine, this aesthetic of return is transposed to a Christian context of grace, in which our own conduct determines our condition both in this life and the next. By the High Middle Ages, Augustinian theologians had mapped out a vigorous theology of knowledge that gave prominence to the mechanical arts and to the role of such arts in restoring in us the divine qualities lost in the Fall. Throughout the later Middle Ages, this view of the mechanical arts survived the rise of Aristotelianism, in which crafts play a servile role, because of the continued prominence of Augustinian theology and of the Austin Canons. In the fourteenth century, the mechanical arts had retained enough of their associations with Christian salvation for *The Siege of Jerusalem* to be able to integrate surgery into its own salutary leitmotif of Christ the Physician. For this poet, surgical treatment is linked implicitly with miraculous expressions of God's grace, in that its goal is to raise the patient above his fallen condition and restore him to the likeness of Christ. This study must remind us, then, that while surgery by its very definition could be associated with fragmentation, pollution, and death, this was not always so—the surgeon fragments, but also reassembles; partitions, but also binds; removes, but also restores. The surgeon both heals and hurts, and in this, he is just like God Himself.

It seems clear that the surgeon, in the mind of the medieval parishioner, could embody both damnation and salvation, and invoke both the integrity of the body as well as its potential for discontinuity. How, we might ask, did performing this profoundly ambivalent art affect the surgeon on the psychic level? How did the surgeon experience his own craft in the face of such contradictory representations? The next two chapters will examine the potential effects of embodying such associations on the literal surgeon and on the priest whose function he symbolizes.

PART II

SURGERY AND EMBODIMENT

CHAPTER 3

THE PRIEST: JOHN AUDELAY'S WOUNDS OF SIN

The surgeon, because he both healed and hurt, served as a uniquely encompassing metaphor for the crucial struggle between damnation and salvation at the heart of medieval Christian identity. The mutilating effects of his violent techniques could suggest the punishments of the damned, as we saw in *Cleanness* and its graphic description of the Dead Sea. Conversely, the physical restoration that resulted from successful treatment reminded authors of the divine grace that attended the bodies of the saved both here and in the afterlife, as *The Siege of Jerusalem* attests. While these two poems help us to understand the importance of the metaphor of the wounds of sin and its treatment, it remains to examine the effects such constructions had on the very men who embodied them: the priest who granted absolution and the surgeon who popularly represented him. This chapter will discuss the first of these figures with reference to the work of John Audelay, whose fifteenth-century single-author anthology of religious verse is doubly valuable as an example of this ubiquitous metaphor and as an autobiographical account of literal affliction and the various cultural meanings that illness assumed in the penitential culture of later medieval England.[1] At the heart of this remarkable collection is an emerging conflict between the physical realities of chronic suffering and the official stance of the Church that confession, because it negates the sins that cause disease, is the only truly efficacious medicine. The overarching narrative in which this conflict plays out in Audelay's anthology can tell us much about both the changing approach to devotion in the fifteenth century and the continued importance of the surgeon to discourses of salvation right up to the eve of the Reformation.

In 1426, Audelay, an aging chantry priest at the Augustinian abbey of Haughmond near Shrewsbury, completed the *Concilium conciencie*, or "þe cownsel of conseans," a unified series of poems on a variety of religious themes.[2] Despite the seclusion of its author and the markedly penitential tone of many of the entries, there remains, in its forays into alliterative style and concern with ecclesiastical governance, an unmistakably worldly aspect to Audelay's remarkable collection. This mixture of voices—the public and sermonic with the private and devotional—is especially pronounced in the longest and most famous poem of the manuscript, "Marcolf and Solomon." In this sprawling verse sermon Audelay adopts the persona of Marcolf, the fool to the paradigmatically wise King Solomon, in order to embark on a trenchant critique of clerical corruption. This rhymed and alliterative work owes more than a passing debt to the reformer spirit and apocalyptic rhetoric of *Piers Plowman*; just as Langland's Will fears that for his decaying England "drede is at the laste," so too does the speaker of Audelay's poem "dred lest dedle sun þis reme wyl deystry."[3] Yet although these two authors are separated by less than half a century, they write their respective volumes under drastically different conditions. This division is not merely centennial but also political. Langland, who died in 1387, writes during an exciting period of religious literature in English, at the peak of what Nicholas Watson has influentially termed "vernacular theology."[4] His attacks on clerical incontinence appear at a historical juncture at which laypeople could participate significantly, even profoundly, in ecclesiastical and doctrinal discussions through an expanding corpus of Middle English religious writing. By contrast, Audelay wrote in the chilly atmosphere that followed the publication of Archbishop Arundel's *Constitutions* in 1409, which sought to counteract the leveling activities of Lollard and orthodox thinkers alike by forbidding authors working in the vernacular from commenting on the sacraments, criticizing the Church, or writing or owning works of even partial scriptural translation without the express consent of an appointed committee.[5] Audelay, according to Richard Firth Green, assumes the Marcolf persona precisely because of "the very danger of speaking too openly," and in James Simpson's words "brilliantly exploits a traditional discursive position."[6]

Yet Audelay is not primarily a political writer but a religious one. His collection as a whole has more in common with the didactic manuals of confession that flowered in the wake of the Fourth Lateran Council than with the overtly political sensibilities of Langland's great poem. Its concerns are largely catechismal, with individual pieces addressing the merits of the Mass, the seven deadly sins, the works of mercy, and the form of general confession. Thus "Marcolf and Solomon," despite its harsh consideration of clerical incontinence, constantly upholds the authority of priests, who alone have the power "to asoyle ȝoue of ȝour synne" (2.802). However, this is also an intensely personal collection. Indeed, it soon becomes apparent that when Audelay adopts the perspective of Marcolf to castigate priests who should be "lanternys of lyf" (2.71) for their "consians vnclere" (2.72), he is equally concerned with his own troubled conscience. A single refrain repeats five times over the course of the *Concilium*, imparting to the reader the information that Audelay, even as he writes and compiles his anthology, suffers from various infirmities as a result of past sins:

> Meruel ȝe noȝt of þis makyng,
> Fore I me excuse hit is not I,
> Fore þis of Godis oun wrytyng
> Þat He send doun fro heuen on hye,
> Fore I couþ neuer bot he foly.
> He haþ me chastist for my leuyng;
> I þonk my God, my Grace treuly,
> Of His gracious vesetyng.
> Beware, serys, I ȝou pray,
> Fore I mad þis with good entent.
> Fore hit is Cristis comawnment;
> Prays fore me þat beþ present,
> My name hit is þe blynd Audelay.
>   (15.196–208)

This "vesetyng" by which God chastises Audelay includes not only sensory impairments but also a seemingly chronic illness; the poet himself tells us on numerous occasions that he is "[d]eeff, siek, blynd" (55.52). Yet despite such frequent assertions, critics are divided on the true extent of Audelay's afflictions and even on whether they can be taken literally at all. At the center of this debate is a tacit insistence on a strict opposition between personal and conventional modes of expression, with commentators viewing Audelay's autobiographical moments as either one or the other type of utterance. Thus Ella Keats Whiting, in her standard edition of the poems, takes Audelay's self-references as evidence that he was literally blind and deaf, but does not confront their potentially metaphorical function.[7] Richard Firth Green also takes the poet at his word, stating as a matter of fact that by the time Audelay completed *Concilium conciencie*, "he was blind, deaf, and sick."[8] Others are more incredulous; for example, Tim William Machan argues that these passages do not in any way "specify the historical John Audelay" but "turn his condition into a metaphor as they come to suggest formulaically that the author of the poem is the prototypical sinner, who is blind and deaf to his own sins and to the salvation of Christ."[9] Eric Stanley, upholding Machan's stance over what he regards as unrealistically romantic appraisals of Audelay's authorial voice, goes even further by insisting that such references do not at all "reveal the poet's inner self" but instead "metaphorize mankind's afflictions of the spirit, as is common in medieval religious verse."[10] Yet as Arthur Kleinman has demonstrated in his classic account of modern illness narratives, it is precisely through the rhetorical conventions of our society that we are able to articulate internal phenomena at all. According to Kleinman, the dominant metanarratives of a culture work to transform the experience of illness from "a wild, disordered natural occurrence into a more or less domesticated, mythologized, ritually controlled, therefore *cultural* experience."[11] As we shall see, the dominant illness narrative of Audelay's time was that of physical affliction as at once both just punishment for sin and merciful remedy for immoderate love of the world. Indeed, there are several reasons to suspect that Audelay's life before his retirement to Haughmond was quite worldly, including a possibly baronial family background and a lively interest in alliterative verse style. Yet the most startling evidence is Audelay's prior membership in the retinue of Lord LeStrange of Knockin, during the course of which he was involved in what Michael Bennett has called "the most notorious act of sacrilege in the kingdom within living memory."[12] In 1417, while attending church in London, LeStrange saw and confronted an enemy, Sir John Trussell. The two were eventually separated only for LeStrange and his squires to return to the church later in the afternoon and attack Trussell in a skirmish that resulted in the violent death of a parishioner who had attempted to make peace between the two parties. Audelay was one of the defendants named in the records of the Court of King's Bench; according to Bennett, the taint of being involved in such a monstrous transgression—the commission of manslaughter in the house of God—drove Audelay to seek the post of chantry priest at Haughmond, soon after which he began to suffer "afflictions which he firmly believed were punishment for his sins."[13]

There is, however, no need to discover a point of origin for Audelay's highly penitential cast of mind.[14] The rhetoric of confession saturated his culture to such an extent that its imagery, metaphors, and tropes necessarily inflected any attempt at self-articulation. As we saw in the introduction chapter of this text, the Fourth Lateran Council of 1215 inaugurated a vibrant tradition of vernacular religious writing on the subject of confession by making mandatory the annual discharge of sins to one's parish priest. Confession was seen as so important to spiritual health that Pope Innocent took the unusual step of ordering this twenty-first canon, the *Omnius utriusque sexus* (everyone of either sex) decree, "frequently published in churches, so that nobody may find the pretence of an excuse in the blindness of ignorance."[15] It quickly became the central operation of the faith and the strict prerequisite to salvation, without which the soul was irrevocably and perpetually damned. John Gaytryge, writing in 1357, presents his entire translation of the broad Latin catechism of Archbishop Thoresby of York as an exposition on "how scrifte es to be made and whareof and in how many thingez solde be consederide."[16] Indeed, we must imagine that the sacrament of confession formed a huge part of the psychological furniture of later medieval parishioners. As Marjorie Curry Woods and Rita Copeland have demonstrated, Christian treatises on confession had by the fourteenth and fifteenth centuries practically replaced classical books as texts in England's increasingly common public schools; and adult confession, because it both began and ended with review of the catechism, was itself a return to the classroom.[17] Children also learned the rhetoric of confession at home from their parents, who were constantly admonished to teach the Christian faith to their sons and daughters. Gaytryge, for example, orders parents who have gained knowledge of essential points of doctrine through the weekly vernacular sermons instituted by Thoresby to "sythen teche tham thair childir, if thay any have, whate tym so thay are of elde to lere tham."[18] This obligation to educate in clerical fashion became an acknowledged part of the duties of parenting. Less than two decades later, *Book to a Mother*, which a country priest in the Southwest Midlands wrote to encourage his widowed mother to adopt a religious life,[19] could lament that "unneþe schullen men finde ony man þat bisiliche techiþ his children fro þe time þat þei konne speke, to drede and worschupe God in holdinge his hestis, and to despise þe world and forsaken hemself and do penaunce."[20] Parents who failed to perform this educating function would eventually find their immortal souls in peril. Indeed, at Judgment Day, according to William Caxton's *Quattuor Sermones*, wayward children will "repreue theyr faders & moders that wold not chastyse them" at the same time as "subgettis accuse theyr euyl curatys that wold not repreue them of theyr synnes ne teche them the commaundementis of God."[21] This conflation of parental and priestly authority, the importance of which I shall address later on in this discussion, found its gestural counterpart in the symbolic action of kneeling. Later medieval tombstone art increasingly depicted the family of the deceased with the children kneeling at the feet of their parents, a prostration that suggested not only intercessory prayer but also virtuous submission to parental authority.[22] For their part, manuals of confession commonly taught penitents to assume a similar posture before the administering parson, as does Audelay himself when he insists that "to þe prest ʒe knele adoune" (17.98). For many of Audelay's contemporaries, then, confession and the catechismal knowledge required to master it was always either at the forefront or dwelling in the margins of their everyday concerns.

Audelay's autobiographical references reflect the cultural primacy of the rhetoric of confession even as the prolonged nature of his illness creates tensions between ecclesiastical claims for the efficacy of penance and the unheeding materiality of the poet's own decaying body. The most common of all rhetorical figures for confession was the metaphor of the wounds of sin. Practically every textbook definition of confession in the fourteenth and fifteenth centuries incorporates this ubiquitous image. The late-fourteenth-century *The Clensyng of Mannes Sowle*, for example, defines confession as "þat þing wherbi a priuy soore or goostli siknesse is opened wiþ hope of forȝeuenesse," while toward the end of our period Caxton's *Quattuor Sermones* describes "a salue sanatyf for alle maner soris of synne when it is dyscretely vsyd."[23] Religious writers frequently encouraged the use of such bodily images because they facilitated the transmission of more challenging, esoteric truths. In his sermon collection *Festial*, for example, Myrk defended the Church's use of icons against Lollard objections by arguing that such "ymages and payntours ben lewde menys bokys."[24] When making such arguments, orthodox writers always hastened to add that images function as aids to contrition rather than as objects of idolatry of the sort prohibited by the First Commandment. Indeed, the fifteenth-century didactic prose work *The Mirroure of the Worlde* insists that in regarding icons "we worshipp not the ymages, for theye be not made alonly but for to brynge to oure mynde the passion that God suffred for vs."[25] Although such discussions tend to refer to representations of Christ and the saints from the plastic arts, Audelay's contemporaries occasionally tackled the question of the legitimacy of imagery from an overtly literary perspective. The Carthusian monk Nicholas Love, whose pseudo-Bonaventurian *Mirror of the Blessed Life of Jesus Christ*, an extremely visual and descriptive guide to affective meditation that was not only immensely popular but also received the official approval of Archbishop Arundel, insists that it is only through imaginative representations of scriptural episodes of the sort he provides that "a symple soule þat kan not þenke bot bodyes or bodily þinges mowe haue somwhat accordynge vnto is affecion where wiþ he maye fede & stire his deuocion."[26] Such creative methods of spurring contrition and spiritual understanding do not distract us from achieving salvation but, according to *Book to a Mother*, formed the basis of Christ's own teaching: Christ, who "wiste wel þat we hadde blend us self and destried oure gostliche wittis," taught the Jews spiritual lessons through "a bodiliche ensample þat þei knewe, for þei shulde þerbi haue knowe gostliche þinges þat he chargede more."[27] Despite the circumscribing effects of Arundel's *Constitutions*, "one of the most draconian pieces of censorship in English history,"[28] religious writers of Audelay's day continued to make central use of the "bodiliche ensample" of the wounds of sin so popular in the previous century. Many of the most influential fourteenth-century religious works not only continued to circulate long after the effects of the *Constitutions* had waned but also enjoyed greater popularity in the fifteenth century than most of the works composed under the crusading archbishop's oversight.[29] The result was that in Audelay's day the wounds of sin remained a vitally important metaphor.

Yet for Audelay, as for his contemporaries, the relationship between physical and spiritual affliction was by no means purely figurative. Indeed, religious writers had long suspected a direct relationship between bodily ailments and moral intemperance. When Innocent, in his famous canon, presented confession as a surgical operation in which the priest must "pour wine over the wounds of the injured one," his purpose was not merely to illustrate the urgency of full confession by way of earthly comparison but also to anticipate the ruling, in the very next canon, that because "sickness of the body may sometimes be the result of sin," patients must send for priests before physicians, "for when the cause ceases so does the effect."[30] So strong was this perceived connection between sin and sickness that subsequent writers invariably adapted Innocent's imagery of wounds and their treatment throughout the later Middle Ages. One such work, *The Middle English "Mirror,"* translated from an earlier Anglo-Norman sermon collection, shows the influence of Innocent's two successive canons by incorporating both registers, the metaphorical and the literal, into its discussions of the wounds of sin. According to the anonymous author, an unconfessed sin is akin to the "wounde þat is heled wiþowten & roteþ wiþynnen & draweþ to þe deþward."[31] Such a formulation refers to the surgical commonplace that incomplete purgation of a wound worsens the problem by trapping corrupt humors inside the orifice. These wounds, according to Roger of Parma, "ben worsse than they were in the first begynnyng."[32] Yet elsewhere in the collection this relationship transcends the merely metaphorical. In keeping with Innocent's justification for the privileging of spiritual over earthly medicine, *The Middle English "Mirror"* insists that internal guilt is often the primary cause of external malady. There were three theories that circulated as to the precise mechanism by which sin led to sickness. The first and most common theory is that God uses illness as a moral corrective, to which Roger of Parma himself subscribes when he states that "god sendeth both good men and yuyl men dyuers syknes both for her own profite and for other mennys prophite and heleth hem aftyrward."[33] The second theory, similar to the first, is that God permits some fulfillment of purgatory here on earth, as when the popular early-fifteenth-century *ars moriendi* treatise *The Crafte of Dying* states that "sekenes before a mannes dethe ys a purgatory to hym when hit ys suffred as hit ought."[34] There was, however, a third, more physiological theory that held that the very real exertion involved in immoral activity causes the humors themselves to gather and corrupt in a single location on the body, leading directly to the formation of a wound. It is precisely for this reason that an anonymous surgeon writing in London at the end of the fourteenth century cautions against lechery, which can "meuen þe humouris, whos cours drawiþ to þe wounde & makiþ it empostime & discrasen."[35] Similarly, according to

The Mirroure of the Worlde, for those who sin regularly "þe flesch is þan in gret flux," and as a result "þe synnes is bitokned be þe flesch that makeþ þe man feble to God."[36] Wounds, then, stood as the literal matter of sin inscribed upon the flesh and were understood as such by both the surgeons who treated them and the religious writers who appropriated them for their discussions of the vices and virtues. We might therefore answer the argument that Audelay's autobiographical references cannot suggest genuine self-reflection but only the obligatory conventions of his time with the observation that our poet could not have helped but view his afflictions in the same penitential framework as was prescribed for the sick across his culture.

The imagery of the wounds of sin is central to Audelay's "Marcolf and Solomon." The real message of this poem, despite its somewhat hackneyed rehearsal of the litany of transgressions of which the clergy was commonly accused, is that priests are absolutely indispensable to the pursuit of salvation, and their authority is unimpeachable. Remarkably, Audelay conveys this discursive denouement in the form of an extended medical metaphor that, although long, is worth quoting in full:

Dredles vche dedly sunne Y declare a wounde,
þat when þe fend haþ foȝt with ȝoue and haþ þe maystre,
þen most ȝe seche a surgoun ȝif ȝe wyl be saue and sound,
þat con soþle serche ȝour sore and make ȝoue hole.
Confession and contresion þi salue schal hit be,
þe penans of þi penetawnsere þi satisfaccion;
þen feȝtust with þe fynd aȝayne and hast þe maystre,
And dost hym schenchip and schame, fore euer confucyon,
þi soule fore to saue.
þus þi woundis helyd schul be
With gret worchip to þe;
Because of þi victore,
Reward schalt þou haue.

Misere mei, Deus, *quia infirmus sum*.

I lekyn vche a synful soule to a seke mon
þat is y-schakyd and schent with þe aksis;
þer is no dayntet e-dyȝt þat pay hym þai con,
Bot al þat is aȝayns hym þat wyl hym pleese;
So hit farus by a mon þat ys recheles,
þat is seke in his soule, þe soþ he nel not here,
Bot wrys away fro Godys word to his wyckydnes;
Here may ȝe know kyndle ȝif ȝour consians be clere,
þe soþ verament.
Cristyn men ȝif þat ȝe be,
þen loke ȝe done cristynle,

Ellus ʒe berun þat nome in veyne, treuly;
ʒe wyl be shamed and y-shent.

(2.897–922)

These two stanzas impart Audelay's ultimately orthodox message by comparing the urgency of confession to that of surgical treatment, and the total authority of the priest over matters of the soul to the surgeon's over those of the body. This comparison is, of course, utterly conventional. The fifteenth-century priest Richard Eremyte, in his commentary on the *Pater Noster*, complains that the typical man of his day "wole suffre of to smyte honde and foot at þe biddyng of his leche," and yet "for his soule heele a litil penaunce wol not vndirtake."[37] Yet Audelay's passage is particularly interesting for its detailed separation of surgeons and physicians, which, as we have seen, resulted historically from Innocent's prohibition against higher orders of clergy shedding blood. In this changed medical context, the surgeon took control of the outside of the body, treating the wounds and other disturbances that marred its surface, while the physician regulated the complex interplay of humors within. This later medieval division between surgeon and physician finds convenient expression in the *Liber Niger*, the household book of Edward IV, in which the duties of the "Mastyr Surgeoune" include "to make playstyrs for the syke officers of this courte" and to "let blood," while the "physycyan," by contrast, must spot those "infected with leper or pestylence" and advise on "wich dyet is best according, and to tell the nature and operacion of all the metes."[38] Texts designed to educate priests in the various strategies of administering confession from before the Fourth Lateran Council conflated both types of medicine into the single figure of the physician. The early seventh-century *Penitential of Columban*, for example, assigns the physician provenance over both internal and external conditions: "the spiritual physicians ought also to heal with various sorts of treatment the wounds, fevers, transgressions, sorrows, sicknesses and infirmities of souls."[39] Even the *Peniteas Cito*, a school textbook composed only a few years before Innocent's influential canon, depicts the physician as responsible for both kinds of condition: "He does not heal a fever as a wound or a tumor."[40] By the later Middle Ages, however, the fragmentation of the healing arts had the corresponding effect of splitting into two the types of medical metaphor clerical writers could employ. Thus Caxton's *Ryall Booke*, a late translation of the Anglo-Norman *Somme le roi* by the thirteenth-century Friar Laurent, instructs sinners to seek the confessor just as they would the doctor but must distinguish between "the leche" and "the physycyen," since one looks to the former when he "feleth hym self hurte of a wounde" and the latter when he "hath euyll humours in his body."[41] That the surgeon takes over from the physician as the primary metaphor for pastoral intervention is hardly surprising. The capacity of surgery to stand for confession arises in large part from its status as the last resort of medicine, which the surgeon performs and the patient submits to only when other methods have failed. As the thirteenth-century Italian surgeon Theodoric of Cervia explains, "the resources of medicine are three, with which treatments the doctor may attack the causes of diseases: diet, draught and surgery."[42] Confession, like surgery, is not preventative but curative. Indeed, penitents were warned against frivolous use of the sacrament and discouraged from seeking absolution without genuine sins to confess.[43] Those who go to confession therefore already suffer, as the immensely popular fourteenth-century poem *Speculum Vitae* would have it, "seknes of syn."[44] While the "surgoun" of the first stanza is clearly the priest, the implied physician of the second is none other than Jesus Christ, or *Christus Medicus*. Because the "seke mon" of this passage did not accept the virtuous "dayntet e-dyȝt" that Christ prescribes, he is now "y-schakyd and schent" with fever, soon to require the last resort of surgery. In other words, after having failed to control his fallible nature in accordance with Christ's laws he must now expiate his sins at the hands of the confessor or face everlasting damnation. This is not an uncommon conceit; the *Fasciculus Morum*, a fourteenth-century preacher's handbook, argues that Christ acts like a physician when he gives the penitent "a diet as he requires and prescribes what he should eat and what he should avoid," thereby helping him "to avoid the occasions of sin and to seek the occasions for practicing the virtues."[45] Yet it is clear that in choosing between these two figures, the surgeon and the physician, for the most effective metaphor for confession, one that captured both the reality of absolution and the difficulty of achieving it, surgery was foremost in the clerical imagination.

Audelay employs this metaphor not only to demonstrate the importance of confession to the laity but also as a means to address his own tenuous spiritual health. Indeed, the final stanza of "Marcolf and Solomon" unites the sermonic "Y" of the medical passage quoted above with a more personal, subjective "I," thus drawing Audelay in his specificity as subject into the conventional rhetoric of the wounds of sin. This merging of the vertical and the horizontal creates a discursive axis that is at once personal to Audelay and exemplary to his readers: Audelay's articulations of suffering render him a living example of God's chastisement. His resulting meekness is evident in the poem's closing lines, in which Audelay defiantly refuses to atone for his castigation of the clergy because to do so would be to affront an even more daunting authority than Archbishop Arundel:

I nel not wraþ my God at my wetyng,
As God haue merce on me, syr Ion Audlay,

At my most ned.
I reche neuer who hit here,
Weder preest or frere,
For at a fole ȝe may lere,
ȝif ȝe wil take hede.

(2.1007–1013)

This passage is indeed notable for its refusal to capitulate to institutional censorship, but it also suggests that Audelay has more on his mind than the distant possibility of persecution. These lines find Audelay "at his most need," and serious illness seems to me a much more plausible explanation for this admission of hardship than fear of retribution, which in any case would hardly have been so imminent as to explain such an ominous self-assertion. If anything, the theory that Audelay believes that there might be retaliation for his poem only strengthens the notion that his autobiographical moments refer to real conditions. Green argues that for Audelay the threat Arundel embodied was very real; he does not translate or even paraphrase the many scriptural quotations in the anthology, and he even makes ominous references to burning informed by the 1401 statute *De Heretico Comburendo*.[46] Indeed, James Simpson goes so far as to suggest that Audelay "explicitly courts the dangers of anti-Lollard persecution."[47] If this is so, then perhaps his fearlessness was the result of the chronic illness from which he expected to die upon completing the *Concilium*. Whiting proposed that the ending of this book was to be the ending of the manuscript but that Audelay "recovered and wrote much more,"[48] while Green takes the generic final words of the colophon, *cuius anime propicietur deus Amen* (The Lord have mercy on his soul. Amen.), as evidence that the poet was in fact already dead. According to Susanna Fein, however, the continuous copying from one section of the manuscript to the other suggests, along with other evidence, that Audelay remained an authorial though ailing presence throughout the entire compilation process.[49] For Fein, the whole manuscript is an eschatological meditation, an exercise in "thinking upon last things."[50] Amidst these different viewpoints, a common thread is that Audelay was indeed suffering during the writing of his book. The tone of the conclusion to "Marcolf and Solomon," with its plain disregard for ecclesiastical retribution, is therefore not one of heroism, as some might romantically wish, but rather resignation—Audelay, increasingly "deeff, siek, blynd," will soon be in the court of a higher judge.

Audelay's afflictions clearly dictated his choices as compiler during the writing of the *Concilium*. The most obvious example of this dynamic is the inclusion of *De visitacione infirmorum et consolacione miserorum*, which attempts to reconcile the tensions that existed between Christ's status as the paradigm of love and the harsh yet ubiquitous fact of tribulation. This poem conflates two common genres, the *consolatio* (consolation) and the visitation of the sick, both of which presented physical affliction as issuing directly from God. It is hard not to see in the impersonally didactic lines that follow an echo of the autobiographical refrain that most links the historical John Audelay to the penitential speaker of the *Concilium*:

> Dissyre ʒe not aʒayne Godis wile,
> Bot euer ald ʒou wel apayd,
> What vesetacion He send ʒou tylle,
> Fore His merce in ʒou He wil fulfil
> When tyme is cum at His lykyng:
> Fore wom He louys He chastest wele,
> And saue his soule fro perescheng,
> Fro þe payns of helle.
>
> (11. 106–113)

In this passage, affliction and remission coexist in an uneasy interdependence: at the very same time that Christ heals illness in the spiritual sense he also causes it on the more immediate level of the body. The surgeon could easily accommodate this jarring ambivalence that attended representations of Christ in religious didactic writing. Indeed, the surgeon became an indispensible point of comparison for the seemingly paradoxical operation of divine mercy precisely because of the painful, even dangerous nature of his healing. Other writings on tribulation contemporary with Audelay's version turn on this comparison between God and the newly distinct figure of the surgical practitioner. *The Book of Tribulation*, for example, contains an extended comparison between the purgation of corrupt humors through bloodletting—"bledynge"—and that of corrupt desires from the heart by means of divinely sent tribulation.[51] The author goes on to compare confession, the true medicine for tribulation, with this central operation of surgery: "And right as the man ylete blood hath nede to purge the wicked blood and the good blood to withholde to norisshynge of the body," so, too, should he "purge the wicked blood of synne."[52] *The Crafte of Dying* goes beyond metaphor to argue that even literal sickness depends on confession for its cure when it insists that "a seke man shuld be counseyled and exorted to prouyde and procure hymself hys soule hele by verrey contrycion and confession," citing Innocent's decree as evidence: "For often tymes, as a certeyn decretall sayth, bodyly sekenes commeth of sekenes of the soule," for which reason "the pope, in the same decretall chargeth straytly euery bodyly leche that he yeue no sekeman no bodyly medecyne vnto the tyme that he hath warned and induced hym to seche his spirituall leche."[53] Not only broad treatments of tribulation but also narrow expositions of the *De Visitacione infirmorum*, the literary version of the rite for the

Visitation of the Sick, allude directly to Innocent's "decretall." One later medieval example insists that "þe lawe wolde by ryght iustice þat no leche schulde zeue bodyliche medicyne to a seek man, but zet he were in wille to take goostliche medicyne and to leue þe synne þat woundeth his sowle, schryuyng hym trewliche with good wille to don no moore euyl."[54] The surgeon emerges as an extremely ambivalent figure, denigrated for the earthly healing he performs while exalted by his figurative role in the transmission of institutional law and doctrinal truth. This tension between earthly and spiritual registers resembles Audelay's own situation as a pious chantry priest who suffered real chronic illness in a culture that recognized physical infirmity as evidence of the much more perilous affliction of the soul. Despite these tensions, the penultimate poem of the *Concilium*, an address by Christ to sinful humanity on the subject of confession and the seven deadly sins, insists that if you "schryue ʒoue clene with repentans," then the Savior, in His own words, "wil withdraw my venchaunce" (17.84, 87). The fact that the pious Audelay's illness continues unabated despite his own presumably regular confession suggests an uneasy relationship between the claims of Innocent and subsequent authorities for the curative properties of penance and the grim realities of physical disability. Audelay's own decaying body becomes a site of contestation between the rhetorical truisms and cultural meanings established by centuries of ecclesiastical writing and the intensely personal and chaotic experience of persistent chronic illness.

It is because of this irreconcilable tension that the final poem of the *Concilium* replaces the unstable quid pro quo dynamic seen above, in which Christ withdraws sickness in return for sincere confession, with another, more sustainable illness narrative: physical affliction as punishment. In this poem, Audelay dreams that he intercedes with God on behalf of his sinful race to prevent an impending onslaught of divine vengeance. The loaded opening line, in which Audelay asserts that this last entry serves to "conclud al my makyng" (18.1), suggests not only an author bringing an extended project to a close but also a man at the end of life settling his affairs. Kleinman has argued that the elderly suffering chronic illness feel an almost universal desire to shape their memory of both past and present experience in accordance with the dominant metanarratives of their culture. Indeed, it does seem in this poem that Audelay expresses "the powerful need near the close of life to make sense of key losses by working out the denouement of the narrative of his life's course."[55] This "narrative," according to Kleinman, is unavoidably inflected, even constituted, by the cultural meanings attached to illness at any given time and location, since in all cases "culture fills the space between the immediate embodiment of sickness as physiological process and its mediated (therefore meaning-laden) experience as human phenomenon."[56] In the following stanza, Audelay combines several such meanings and conflates them with the purpose of the *Concilium* as a whole:

> Fore al þat is nedeful to bode and soule
> Here in þis boke þen may ȝe se,
> And take record of þe apostil Poule
> Þat Crist callid to grace and His merce,
> Fore so I hope he haþ done me
> And ȝeuen me wil, wit, tyme, and space,
> Þroȝ þe Hole Gost, blynd, def to be,
> And say þis wordis þroȝ His gret grace.
> So synful a wreche, vnworþely
> Y pray ȝou, seris, fore Cristis sake,
> Ensampil at me þat ȝe take
> And amendis betime ȝe make
> Wile ȝe han space here specialy.
>   (18.14–26)

In this single passage Audelay rationalizes his illness in three distinct ways: as an example to others to reform their lives, as a manifestation of Christ's mercy, and as an early purgatory here in the world, which he later makes explicit by expressing joy that he can "haue my payne, my purgatory / Out of þis word or þat I dy" (18.478–79). As Fein has already noticed, Audelay employs a future construction to describe his ailing condition—"blynd, def *to be*"—and this would seem to suggest that his afflictions continued to develop even as he was completing the *Concilium*.[57] Indeed, an important fact that has been lost in the debate as to whether Audelay could really have been "blynd" while compiling this manuscript is that blindness itself was thought to manifest in various degrees of severity. The Middle English translation of the *De Probatissima Arte Oculorum* of the elusive thirteenth-century medical writer Benvenutus Grassus, for example, attests to a wide range of impairments in cataract patients:

> But nat forþan I perceuyd wele þat of thies maner cateractys were dyuersi-tee, foor sum of them myȝt see the bryȝtnes of the son and went by the way wyth opon ey as thow þei had perfȝtly seyn. And sum myȝte see the stature of a man and of a best or of another thyng and not els. And sum had thys lytle parte of lyȝte to her lyues ende, and of sum yt vanyshyd avaye and þei hade no more syȝte as towe þei neuer had none.[58]

There is, then, a strong possibility that Audelay's own sight steadily and progressively "vanyshyd" rather than abruptly failed. Such a continuing source of despair would help to explain the note of frustration in the poem's penultimate stanza, in which the aging chantry priest, sleepless, unsettled, and "seke in my langure," throws up his hands to God in grim acknowledgment that he needs "[m]ekele to take þi vesetyng / Ellis wot I wil þat I were lorne" (18.482, 489–90). In these lines, it is Christ's vengeance rather than His mercy that Audelay adopts as the context for his suffering. It seems clear that despite Stanley's assertion that "to understand Audelay's lyric art we must not look for personalism,"[59] Audelay does indeed express his own personal experience of suffering the only way he can: through the institutionally sanctioned view of the ailing body as a symbol of penance and by means of the descriptive conventions that constituted the particular limits of articulation available in the England of the fifteenth century.

These limits were, however, expanding even as Audelay was compiling this manuscript. The explosion in Marian veneration that occurred in Audelay's lifetime was part of a larger shift in the devotional landscape that saw the sometimes rigidly doctrinal emphasis of fourteenth-century didactic literature give way to a new interest in emotional responses to sacred history. This interest was spurred in large part by the entry of female visionary writing into England in the last decade of the fourteenth century,[60] most notably that of St. Bridget of Sweden, to whom Audelay dedicates one of the longer poems of the manuscript.[61] Gail MacMurray Gibson has described this emerging affective piety as an "Incarnational Aesthetic," and its main attribute as an earnest, empowering desire to "transform the abstract and theological into the personal and concrete."[62] While the abstract points of catechism remained an important part of Christian devotion, religious writers exhibited "a growing tendency to see the world saturated with sacramental possibility and meaning and to celebrate it."[63] The manner in which Audelay resumes his project after the *Concilium* reflects these cultural developments. The uniformly Christological matter of the *Concilium* gives way in the next section of the manuscript to a series of lyrics celebrating the Virgin Mary, headed by the incipit *Hic incipunt salutaciones beate Marie virginis* (here begin the salutations to the Blessed Virgin Mary).[64] This change from the Trinitarian to the Marian does not seem so abrupt if we consider that Audelay's intercession with God on behalf of humanity in the closing poem of the *Concilium* anticipates the Marian material by appropriating what by the fifteenth century had become Mary's most famous persona: that of *mediatrix*. For the penitent Christian, the Virgin had for the most part replaced the Son as the foremost paragon of mercy. An explanation for this shift in devotional emphasis can be found in the increasing harshness of literary portrayals of Jesus. Innocent's drive to institute annual confession as the central ritual of the faith required for its success that Christ, whose main attribute is boundless love, assume a more intimidating aspect so as to impress upon parishioners the urgency of absolution. By Audelay's day, Christ had long been depicted far too ambivalently to function purely as a merciful or reassuring figure. Indeed, he was increasingly portrayed as the uncompromising judge who at the trumpet's sound would abandon countless of his children to eternal punishment. It was this punitive Christ to whom religious writers often had recourse when encouraging parishioners to confess frequently and die well. The fourteenth-century spiritual guide *Pore Caitif*, for example, insists on the profound transformation by which "crist þat shal be iuge þere is now meke as a lombe & redi to bowe to merci" but on the last day "wole be steern as a lioun to all þat ben dampnable."[65] This intimidating depiction finds fuller, and more terrifying, expression in the religious poem *Speculum Gy de Warewycke*:

> þider he wole come on domesday,
> Cruwel and sterne wid-oute nay,
> He þat was woned to be
> Meke as a lomb, ful of pite:
> þeder he wole lihten adoun
> Wraþfull and sterne as a lioun.
> Merci nele he shewe non,
> Ac, riht after þat man haþ don,
> He shal fonge his iugement
> To ioye or to stronge turment.
> (ll. 257–66)

This judgmental figure required an effective and accessible intercessor with enough spiritual authority to plausibly influence the hand of God. Indeed, throughout the fourteenth and fifteenth centuries Mary was increasingly seen as the diametric opposite of her necessarily stern Son. The late-fourteenth-century Northern poem *Quatrefoil of Love* weaves Mary into the fabric of the Trinity by portraying her as one of four leaves alongside the Father, Son, and Holy Ghost, but warns that her powers of intercession will end at Judgment Day, when "oure lady Marie dare nott for drede/ Speke till hir dere son, so dredfull es he."[66] During this lifetime, however, prayers to Mary can be more efficacious than those directed at God Himself. According to the fifteenth-century *The Prickynge of Love*, a Middle English version of the *Stimulis amoris* of the Franciscan James of Milan, those to whom Christ turns His back can always appeal to Mary: "sheo kan not but mercy & pite. and sheo may not but preie for synneris. sheo is so woned for to helpen alle. þat I hope þat sheo wol not lere now a newe lessoun for me."[67] If Audelay had indeed expected to die after the *Concilium*, this series of lyrics might represent not only another aspect of his concern with "last things," as Fein would have it, but also something more pragmatic: a renewed attempt to seek succor from his condition through a literary appeal to the endlessly merciful Virgin.

Devotional writing in the affective tradition tends not to incorporate the solemn imagery of the wounds of sin or the surgeon who heals them. As a figure of perfect forgiveness, Mary could hardly accommodate the painful associations that necessarily attended the incorporation of surgery into religious discourses. Indeed, the wound itself, without which the surgeon has no metaphorical place at all, transforms in works of affective devotion from a grim specter of sin to a symbol of divine grace. While Richard Rolle's highly affective meditations contain wound imagery, their medical context is not the invasive surgery of the confessional manuals but the more gentle, second part of medicine: the application of healing herbs. As Rolle claims in his address to Christ, "þy body is lyk to a medew ful of swete flours and holsome herbes: so in þy body fulle of woundes swet sauorynge to a deuout soule, and holsome as herbes to euch synful man."[68] The image of the wound thus becomes a means to transcend sin rather than the literal manifestation thereof, reflecting the tendency of fifteenth-century religious writers to privilege the reassuringly salutary over the grimly cautionary. Similarly, the anonymous author of the popular fourteenth-century lyric "An Autumn Song" compares Mary's intercessions to the physician's soothing treatment through herbal medicines. Like the Christ of Rolle's lines, Mary heals not through the traumatic violence of surgery but rather through the painless apothecary's craft:

> [W]e shulen in-to heuene blis
> þurh hire medicine.
> betere is hire medycyn
> þen eny mede or eny wyn—
> hire herbes smulleþ suete—
> from catenas in-to deuelyn
> nis þer no leche so fyn
> oure serewes to bete.[69]

Yet the figure of the surgeon had accrued too much force as a symbol of penance for Mary to remain completely unaffected by this culturally ubiquitous metaphor. Although Mary is nowhere in the lyric tradition associated with practical medicine, she can be found in the guise of a trained surgeon in another, more unlikely source: Middle English romance. Religious writers defined romance as a dangerously secular genre, sometimes incorporating it directly into descriptions of the various deadly sins. *The Clensyng of Mannes Sowle*, for example, contains a sample confession for sloth in which the hypothetical sinner admits that he has "red on romauncis and fablis and songis and carollis of dishoneste and synne and nycetees."[70] More famously, the *Speculum Vitae* establishes its austere tone and spiritual intent with the opening announcement that its author "wille make ne vayn carpynge" of Bevis of Hampton, Octavian, Ysumbras, or, in fact, anything to do with "dedes of armys."[71] So entrenched was this clerical disdain for romance that the anonymous author of *The Middle English "Mirror,"* convinced that readers of such tales are guilty of "more þen ydelschyp" but "trespaseþ gretlyche," begins writing precisely because of the pressing need to replace secular reading with the kind of edifying matter by which "þe soule may be comforted."[72] Yet for many readers, romance clearly did comfort the soul. As Roger Dalrymple has shown, the highly generic pious tags prevalent in even the most secular romances "figure the salient episodes of salvation history," binding readers across various geographical locations into an implied community of the faithful.[73] Not only intrinsic evidence, but also household manuscripts in which pastoral, devotional, and romance works meaningfully coexist suggest that the laity did not share this negative view of romance as a frivolous, purely secular form of literature. Through romance, the surgeon acquired an entirely different connotation than was possible in strictly didactic religious writings.

The female healer of romance was sometimes not only a surgeon but also an imaginative figure for the Virgin Mary. Through such representations, the metaphor of the surgeon marched in lockstep with the changing nature of devotional practice. The comforting imagery of the female romance healer dilutes the unsettling descriptions of surgery common to penitential contexts in much the same way that the reassuring magnanimity of Mary removes the sting from the terrifying Christ of Judgment Day. Almost always a courtly lady, she often appears under mysterious circumstances in the presence of her handmaidens to heal an injured knight. The depth of medical detail is occasionally quite profound, as is the case with John Lydgate's *The Siege of Thebes*. This passage, although not explicitly Marian in the manner of the example to follow, demonstrates the wide range of medical knowledge attributed to the female healer in medieval romance:

> And first this lady / of her wommanhede
> Hir wymmen badde / as goodly as they kan,
> To be attendaunt on this wounded man.
> And whan he was vnarmed to his scherte,
> She made first wassh his woundes smerte,
> And serche hem wel / with dyuers instrumentes,
> And made fette / sondry oynementes,
> And leches ek / the beste she koude fynde,

Ful craftely to staunche hem / and to bynde,
And euery thing / that may do him ease
Taswage his peyn / or his woo tapese,
Was in the courte / and in the Castel sought,
And by her byddyng / to his chambre brought.
And for his sake / she hath after sent
For swich deyntees / as wern conuenyent,
Moost nutrityf / be phisikes lore,
Hem that wern syk / or wounded / to restore[74]

This scene, in which Lygurge's daughter heals the wounded hero, is not overtly Marian but is remarkable for its realistic portrayal of medieval wound treatment, which always began with careful diagnosis. This is a crucial step, as wounds could have different humoral characteristics, and the variety of ointment the educated surgeon applied depended on the specific wound's particular humoral properties. The important thing was to ensure that the salve contained contrary attributes to the superfluities found in the wound itself, so as to negate any fatal excesses and restore balance to the limb. The use of the word "serche" to describe either the visual or manual diagnosis of a wound conforms to the language used in Middle English translations of surgical texts, such as when William of Saliceto attributes surgical accidents to an "ignoraunce of serchynge."[75] Afterward she prescribes a dietary regimen according to "phisikes lore," as surgeons frequently did in order to protect the delicate humoral balance their treatments restored and prevent any dangerous relapse. Our anonymous London surgeon, for example, insists that patients suffering from head wounds "schal ete no fisch, ne eggis, ne almaunde-mylk, ne noon oþir mylk, ne þou schalt not ete no maner fruit," each of which "engendriþ corrupcioun and empostymeþ the wounde, and bringiþ þe sike man to his deeþe."[76] Lydgate's lines exemplify just how developed the romance convention of the female healer had become by the fifteenth century. It is for this reason that Muriel Joy Hughes, in her monograph on this enigmatic figure published in the middle of the last century, approached the subject purely from the perspective of medical history.[77] Despite the impressive amount of medical detail she unearths, Hughes neglects to consider the religious resonances of the romance healer. As the sprawling fifteenth-century romance *Eger and Grime* demonstrates, this mysterious lady's gestures and appearance often resemble to a large extent the newly central personage of the Virgin Mary.

Eger and Grime contains a particularly rich example of the Marian romance healer.[78] In the scene in question, the hero Sir Eger lies wounded after battling with a notorious knight in an ill-advised attempt to impress the beautiful Winglayne, when suddenly a courtly lady emerges from a castle garden flanked by two handmaidens. Marian associations abound in the extended description of healing that follows. According to Eger, Loosepaine is "cladd in scarlett redd" with skin "red as rose," an attribute that accords with the popular image of Mary as *Rosa Mystica* depicted most famously in Van der Weyden's well-known painting of the "Virgin and Child."[79] The handmaidens, too, suggest Mary in their unavoidable resemblance to the apocryphal handmaidens of Christ, Salome and Zelomi, in the *Protevanegelium* of James. Just as these two women were frequently depicted in medieval art washing Christ in a basin, so too do the handmaidens of *Eger and Grime* take part in a similarly baptismal scene by washing the wounded knight in a "siluer bason" (l. 251). After the healing itself, during which, according to Eger, Loosepaine "searched my woundes" (l. 246), the three ladies sing to the accompaniment of a harp. The harp was the well-known symbol of the Old Testament King David,[80] who used its soothing tones to heal the possessed monarch King Saul. Because Mary was popularly considered to be David's direct descendant, the harp of this scene suggests the unification of the Old and New Laws that Mary embodied, as well as the universal healing of the sins of Adam made possible by the Incarnation. Indeed, the poet communicates the solemnly religious nature of this episode as a whole by transforming it into a scene of *pietas*, in which "oft the weeped, and their hands wrange" before the wounded hero (l. 372). This detail, embedded in such an overtly Marian tableau, would by Audelay's day have assumed great affective force. Indeed, fifteenth-century devotional guides frequently encouraged heavy weeping as a means to elicit Mary's support. *A Devout Treatise Called the Tree and the Twelve Frutes of the Holy Ghost* insists that an essential component of "meditatif prayer is þat it is desirous bi weyling, sobbyng, and syghyng," a methodology the speaker of *The Prickynge of Love* embraces when he confesses that "myne y3en wepen sum-tyme whenne i speke to þis lady."[81] Mary's role as the new paradigm of mercy unimpeded by an Old Testament ethos of justice allows for an affective reformulation of the surgical metaphor. Far from the punitive corrector come to negate the wounds of sin, the surgeon of *Eger and Grime* is the thoroughly nurturing maternal healer.[82] Nor is the wound itself the very sign of transgression against God, but rather a symbol of affinity with Christ's own sacrificial humanity. It is no wonder, then, that after the disappointments of *Christus Medicus* Audelay should instead turn to Mary as "medicyn of al our syne" (19.62) and "medycyne þat ale may mend" (20.101).

Despite this detour into Marian veneration, Audelay soon returns to the profoundly penitential discourse of the first section of the manuscript. The poem *Cantalena de puerica*, an anomalous celebration of the virtues of children, appears after an extended series of jubilant carols completely free of the penitential references to illness that unite the poems of the *Concilium*. In the final stanza of the *Cantalena*, however, Audelay reverts to his earlier assertion that his suffering amounts to an early purgatory:

> Now oþer cumford se I non
> Bot schryue me clene with contricion,
> And make here trew satisfaccion,
> And do my penans wyle Y am here.
>   (41.31–34)

In spite of the apparent inefficacy of confession to heal his sickness, Audelay continues to assert the dominant illness narrative affirmed by both the Fourth Lateran Council and the didactic writings it inspired: that physical affliction not only betokens but in fact derives from unexpiated sin. The imagery of the afflicted body was so endemic to descriptions of the vices and virtues that the sick could not help but internalize this penitential commonplace. The psychologist Henry Laughlin has described the process by which we incorporate cultural attitudes into our experience of self as the "mental mechanism operating outside of and beyond conscious awareness through which external attributes, attitudes, or standards are, or have been, taken within oneself, that is, internalized."[83] In later medieval England, such "external attributes" derived from the didactic literature of confession and the urgent struggle between damnation and salvation it described. The battleground on which this struggle took place was the imagination itself. Indeed, *A Myrour to Lewde Men and Wymmen*, a fifteenth-century prose version of the *Speculum Vitae*, defines sin as the progress from imagination to determination, a fourfold process in which the first step "is in þoght, þe secounde in delyt, þe þridde in consentynge of wille, and þe ferþe in desire to fulfille it in dede."[84] Although mere thought constitutes only a venial sin, extended consideration of the object of desire leads to "delite, and þat may be dedly synne ȝif þe herte longe abyde þerynne."[85] In this fashion, according to Caxton's *Doctrinal of Sapience*, "no synne is venyal but it may be mortal, þat is to saye, whan a persone hath therin playsance and delectacyon."[86] There is, then, a certain circularity to confession. Just as relapse into deadly sin was both frequent and inevitable, so too was the renewed internalization of the wounded and sullied self-image central to sermonic, prosaic, and poetic discussions of spiritual transgression. We can imagine that Audelay, whose ailing body already signaled moral corruption, was particularly prone to such internalization.

In the *Cantalena* Audelay seems to acknowledge this circularity. In the bulk of the poem, he longingly envisions a state of childhood free from moral intemperance, an idealized depiction of youth that Whiting has already noticed departs significantly from the conventionally negative view of childhood found in penitential writing:

> And God wold graunt me my prayer,
> A child aȝene I wolde I were.
> Fore pride in herte he hatis all one;
> Worchip ne reuerens kepis he non;
> Ne he is wroþ with no mon;
> In charete is alle his chere.
>
> (41.1–6)

This sanctification of the young, according to Whiting, "reminds one of the attitude of poets of a later age, and was, indeed, most unusual in Audelay's time."[87] Indeed, as we shall see, didactic writings tended to depict children as precisely the opposite of Audelay's idealized, charitable subjects. Perhaps the point, then, is not that children are truly pristine in their behavior but that the Christian before the age of discretion is not responsible for his or her transgressions. Free from guilt, the child is also free from the crippling anxieties that come with embodying the wounded sinner of penitential discourse. Significantly, medical imagery of the sort Audelay employed in "Marcolf and Solomon" almost always occurs in close proximity to, and even within, penitential metaphors of childhood and parental discipline. Such metaphors act in concert with our earliest, supremely ambivalent experiences of parental power to strengthen the authority of the clergy. The vast influence the rhetoric of confession exercised over authors of Middle English poetry and prose derived from the psychological power of these constantly reiterated familial images, which Audelay and his contemporaries internalized through the interpersonal phenomenon that Freud labeled "transference."

Transference is the concluding phase of psychoanalytic therapy, in which "the patient sees in his analyst the return—the reincarnation—of some important figure out of his childhood or past, and consequently transfers onto him feelings and reactions that undoubtedly applied to this model."[88] By inserting themselves into the unfolding narrative of an analysis, therapists, otherwise powerless to provoke from patients the traumatic confessions necessary to achieve catharsis, assume the role of parental authorities. Freud, having found that all power is experienced as a reformulation of the parental, aggressively positioned himself as a father figure in this way so that he could elicit admissions "which in the real world seem scarcely possible."[89] Similarly, the parish priest, in keeping with the extensive literature of penance and pastoral care available to him, encourages the penitent to associate the confessional interview with his earliest experiences of parental handling and authority. Indeed, so intimate is the relationship between confessor and confessant and so strong its potential for transference that even today therapists fear that when their patients go to confession, "a new relationship with a new therapist will be established, that the transference will be split and a part of it taken away from the psychotherapist and given over to the priest who hears confession."[90] Through ubiquitous comparisons of the confessor to a mother, father, or schoolmaster, and their rearticulation by the administering parson, the penitent learned to connect the parish priest to his most important internalized objects. Because such objects are crucial to the formation of the conscience, the grounds of socialization, they are necessarily disciplinary, and contain harsh affects. Confession, of course, depends for its power on the strength of the individual conscience. As Myrk insists, "þat man þat haþe don a dedly synne, yif he schall be sauved, he schall never take rest yn hys concyens, tyll he be schryven of."[91] According to the Freudian revisionist Heinz Kohut, conscience itself is explicitly parental in origin: "Patients have unconscious presences of actual parental emotional attitudes that wield enormous influences on their lives."[92] In penitential literature, three sets of conventional images work to activate these "unconscious presences": the excremental, the paternal, and the maternal.

One of the most frequent penitential images is that of excrement. The metaphor of sin as feces, vomit, and other impure substances recalls—indeed, reactivates—the anxieties of our earliest indoctrination into the difference between right and wrong, acceptable and unacceptable. Although the association between excrement and moral transgression is an ancient one, it was best known to the Middle Ages in the form of St. Bernard's remedy against pride, which encouraged penitents to contemplate the essentially fecal nature of the human body. Caxton, toward the end of our period, paraphrases this Bernardine notion in his *Doctrinal of Sapience*:

> Seint Bernard saith that who shold wel beholde & take hede of that whiche yssueth out of the eyes, of the eres, of the nosthrillis, of the mouth, of the heeris, of the nailles or vngles of hondes, of feet, & of all other conduites of all the body & of all the flessh, he shold finde that ther is non so vyle ne so stinkyng as is that which issueth & cometh out of the bodyes of men & of wymen, & as we be oueral the body foul hooly.[93]

This sentiment was widely expressed throughout the later medieval period, and rendered the orifices of the body points of extreme anxiety. Indeed, the body's surface is always already a source of tension, at least on an unconscious level. According to Freud, toilet training is the point at which we first come to experience the parents, and the external world they represent, as an inhibiting force: "An infant must not produce his excreta at whatever moment he chooses, but when other people decide that he shall."[94] Julia Kristeva expands Freud's argument to suggest that the mastery of such production is our earliest indoctrination into the binary logic of selfhood, in which bodily residues "stand for the danger to identity that comes from without: the ego threatened by the non-ego, society threatened by its outside, life by death."[95] It is therefore not surprising that we so frequently find such comparisons of sin to excrement in penitential contexts. The superfluities of the body—the very matter of sin, according to Bernard—delineate the boundaries between permissible and impermissible behavior. The thirteenth-century *Ancrene Wisse*, our earliest Middle English pastoral manual, contains many such Bernardine references comparing physical beauty to excrement, for example: "In the middle of the glory of your face, which is your most beautiful part, between the mouth's taste and the nose's smell, do you not bear two toilet holes, as it were?"[96] Although the existence of such literary tropes does not itself prove that the act of confession contained such imagery, the genre of *forma confitendi*, verse templates designed to help parishioners discharge their sins to the priest, suggests that the language of excrement was in fact present in the confessional interview. One of the more popular examples, "St. Brendan's Confession," contains the following admission: "I haue also, my lorde God, behiȝt to þe and to þe preeste, to leue and to forsake synne and algatis ȝet I dwelle and walter þerynne as a fat sowe in hoot somere, turnynge and wendiþ hur in þe foule, stynkyng slow."[97] Sinners, it seems, were actively encouraged to regard themselves as sullied by their transgressions, a self-representation unavoidably connected to our most fraught period of personality development. Melanie Klein, a pioneer of child psychology, saw in these early years of life the primitive beginnings of conscience: "the frequent nightmares and phobias of young children derive from the terror of persecutory parents who by internalization form the basis of the relentless superego."[98] It is to these "persecutory" figures that we now turn.

The father looms large in Middle English religious prose. Most often, he serves as a metaphor by which to explain an enduring tension in Christian theology: the fact of tribulation. Like God, the loving father disciplines his children with necessary severity. Much of the power of this metaphor derives from the apparent consensus in the medieval period that physical discipline is integral to raising obedient children. One popular fourteenth-century poem on parenting insists on the following:

> In children were is now mirþe & now debate,
> In her quarel is no violence,
> Now pleie, now wepinge, & seelde in oon state;
> To her pleyntis ȝeue no credence;
> A rodde reformeþ al her necgligence;

in her corage no rancour dooþ abide,
who þat spariþ þe rodde all vertues settiþ a-side.[99]

Unlike Audelay, this anonymous poet constructs youth as a state of uncontrollable desire requiring the correction of physical force, here imaged as the "rodde" of discipline. In the case of the children of wealthier parents, the schoolmaster frequently stood in as corrector. John Drury, a Suffolk schoolmaster of the fifteenth century, certainly suggests as much when he writes the following practice sentence for his young pupils: "Myn ars comyng to scole xal be betyn."[100] God by no means spares the rod in correcting such solipsism in his own children. Such metaphors of corporeal punishment are especially strong in the textual tradition based on *Somme le roi*, the influential Anglo-Norman manual of confession composed in the thirteenth century. The *Ayenbite of Inwit*, for example, describes sin as a form of childish regression: gluttons are "ase is þet child þet wyle alneway habbe þet bread ine his hand," the prideful "ase is þet child þet loueþ more an sseawere þanne ane kingdome," and the slothful, "ase þet child þet is echedaye beuore his maistre and naȝt can his lessoun."[101] This construction of children is not purely rhetorical. Psychologists often refer to early childhood as a period of "primary narcissism," a solipsistic stage in which the child experiences his body as part of the mother, a closed economy of desire and gratification, and has yet to invest affectively in the external world. In their expositions on the *Pater Noster* and the Fourth Commandment, pastoral writers found ample opportunity to suggest means to correct such narcissism in their spiritual children. According to *The Mirroure for Lewde Men and Wymmen*, the parents of the Fourth Commandment include not only our biological caregivers, "þat is to seie thi fader and thi moder bodiliche," but also "thi fader and moder gostliche, þat is to seie thi gostliche fader þat haþ cure of thi soule and þi moder Holi Chirche."[102] This conventional projection of parental power onto the priest associates confession with our most formative experiences of authority. Similarly, *The Book of Vices and Virtues*, the most literal translation of the *Somme le roi*, states in its exposition on the *Pater Noster* that God "beteþ hem and chasteþ hem whan þei mysdoþ, for here owne profitt, as a good fadre, and gladly receyueþ hem whan þei comeþ to hym."[103] These parallel conflations of God with father and parishioner with child function not only as metaphor but also serve to heighten the emotional properties of confession by encouraging the conflation of parental and clerical authority.

The mother too appears in the literature as an ambivalent, disciplinary figure, but she does so with a great deal more tension and complexity than the father. The mother, unlike the father, is tainted with the very filth she controls in her children. The pseudo-Rollean *Myror of Synneres* urges us to combat pride by reflecting on "how vile a mater þow woxe vp in thy modris wombe," an absolutely conventional sentiment expressed even more venomously in *The Mirroure of the World*, which urges the reader to consider not only "the fylthe of his concepcion" but also that of his own body, "a sakke fulle of mire and of dunge."[104] Yet in Caxton's *Quattuor Sermones*, the mother easily replaces the father as the figurative placeholder for God's own disciplining authority: "As the diere moder chastyseth her childe for takyng of harme when it nygheth fyre or water, right so the fader of heuen chastyseth the to be waar of fleyng away."[105] Indeed, in *A Myrour to Lewde Men and Wymmen*, the tribulations God sends us are not those of a disciplining father at all, but rather "þe ʒerde of þe moder þat chastiseþ her child."[106] We might reconcile these opposing constructions of maternity by noting that maternal authority is always bound up with excremental associations; it is traditionally the mother, and not the father, who acts as "the trustee of that mapping of the self's clean and proper body."[107] This ambivalence also makes sense if we consider the child's intensely symbiotic relationship with the mother in the first two years of life, a unity so pronounced that Donald D. Winnicott, a pioneer of developmental psychology, can insist that "there is no such thing as a baby."[108] According to Winnicott, the child develops a sense of autonomy only through his involvement in such transitional activities as the familiar "peekaboo" game, by which he learns that the mother's terrifying absences are always only temporary. Significantly, we find just such a game represented in *The Chastising of God's Children*. Here, the anonymous author compares God's occasional removal of grace from our lives to "a louynge modir þat listeþ to pley wiþ hir sowkynge child, whiche modir in hir pley sumtyme hideþ hir, and comeþ aʒen to knowe bi þe countenaunce of þe child how wele it loueþ þe modir."[109] Such "pley," we now know, serves the important purpose of educating the child in the disappointments of the external world. Remarkably, the author seems aware of this developmental function, depicting the lovely game as continuous with later, more violent lessons. As the child grows, becoming wiser and stronger, the mother "wiþdraweþ hir glad chiere and sumtyme spekiþ sharpli, sumtyme þreteneþ him, and if þe childe wex wanton, she betiþ him," in the same way that God "chastiseþ whom he loueþ."[110] As with the father, then, the sinner learns to associate this figurative mother with painful discipline and to accept this discipline as an aspect of the tribulation that more than any other experience defines this earthly thoroughfare.

The surgeon was absorbed directly into this interpersonal matrix. As the liaison psychiatrist John Fleming notes, the modern surgeon, "by directly supporting the beleaguered ego, psychologically becomes a transference figure: a parent to a childlike patient."[111] This was as true of the Middle

Ages as it is today. The surgeon's direct handling of the body conflates him not only with the confessor, but also with the parental representations that abound in pastoral literature. *The Chastising of God's Children*, for example, has father and surgeon one and the same: "he smyteþ þat he may heele, and betiþ outward þat he may heele inward þe woundis of trespassis."[112] This association is more overtly rendered in the *Visitatio infirmorum*, which warns that those who complain of fatal illness "greuest thi fadir þe whiche coueiteth to be thi leche."[113] John Trevisa, in his translation of Bartholomaeus Anglicus's thirteenth-century encyclopedia *De proprietatibus rerum*, stressed the fact that the defining attribute of the surgeon is that he does not stop "keruynge oþir brennynge for wepinge of þe pacient."[114] It is precisely this uncompromising quality that the fourteenth-century Augustinian Canon William of Shoreham, in his poem on the seven sacraments, attributed to the ideal priest:

> ȝet he þe schal anoye aȝt,
> Hyt wyle of-þenche hym sore;
> And oþer-wyl anoye he mot,
> Wanne he scheweþ þe lore of helþe,
> Ase mot þe leche ine uoule sores,
> Wanne he royneþ þe felþe.[115]

The priest, the surgeon, and the parent must each clean the "felþe" from their charges and restore them to purity. Through these interlocking metaphors the parishioner comes to internalize both kinds of healer, the spiritual and the physical, as parental figures and to see themselves as children sullied and wounded by sin.

Audelay's book stands as an excellent example of this gradual internalization. Indeed, it is his own status as "felþe" that he most prominently invokes as his work as a whole draws to a close. At the beginning of the anthology, in *De effusione sanguinis Christi*, Audelay engaged impersonally in the sort of excremental rhetoric described above, calling lechery "þat stynkyng syn" and warning his readers to "neuer in slouþ stynke" (4.23, 52). Now, in one of the last poems in the collection, his take on the popular *Timor mortis conturbat me* tradition, Audelay again incorporates this convention but, in a startling admission of penitential self-loathing, applies it directly to himself:

> Here is a cause of gret mornynge;
> Of myselfe no þyng I se,
> Saue filþ, vnclennes, vile stynkyng;
> *Passio Christi conforta me.*
> (51.19–22)

Audelay, far from approximating the childlike innocence of the *Cantalena*, reaches a new nadir of self-admonishment in this description of his own corruption, a tone perhaps attributable to his continued illness, which in its very persistence signals his spiritual impurity and failure of atonement. Indeed, despite his many prayers he even now lies deaf, blind, and "seke in my body" (51.12). From this perspective, we can glimpse Audelay's despair at the unraveling of his illness narrative—his failure to find relief from his afflictions through either the healing properties of confession or the intercessory powers of Mary—in the pattern of spiraling pleas for mediation that have occurred throughout the anthology. Indeed, he has prayed for Christ to intercede with God, Mary to intercede with Christ, and then, in *De Sanctu Anna matre Marie*, for St. Anne to intercede with Mary, "oure soulis leche" (43.2, 5). He is at one remove after another from the original illness narrative of the *Concilium*, after which *Christus Medicus* was to deliver him from this thoroughfare of woe and give meaning to his earthly suffering. Now, after his many prayers to Mary and the various saints, and perhaps even more certain of an impending death, Audelay again returns to the "midsyne" of the "v woundis of Ihesu Crist" (51.27–28). Ultimately, however, a more touching narrative asserts itself. In the anthology's final poem, the afflicted poet suggests that it is ultimately his example to others that gives meaning to all that he has suffered, a salutary gift to the world that, to Audelay, might constitute the real purpose of a dotage marred by sin and prolonged by apparently ineffective atonement:

> Herefore Y haue dyspysed þis worlde
> And haue ouercomen alle ertheley þyng;
> My ryches in heuen with dede and worde
> I haue y-purchest in my leuyng,
> With good ensampul to odur ȝefyng.
>   (55.27–31)

While these lines impart a sense of calm resignation, it is hardly reassuring to think that despite the ministrations of the spiritual "surgoun"—the confessor who promises health of body and of soul—Audelay remains, in his closing words, "Deef, siek, blynd as he lay." In the book of John Audelay, then, we discern another layer of tension in the surgical metaphor: its inevitable failure to sustain itself in the face of the painful and unstoppable progress of literal physical affliction. Audelay therefore provides us with a valuable glimpse into the psychology not only of the priest who occupies the literal half of the metaphor of the surgeon-confessor but also of the patient whose own afflicted body must stand as a symbol for the perils of spiritual transgression. Kleinman notes that in the experience of illness, "cultural meanings mark the sick person, stamping him or her with significance often unwanted and neither easily warded off nor coped with."[116] While it is true that Audelay does not cope easily with his afflictions, he does somewhat transcend them by writing a book that holds up his wounded, sinful body as an example to all, at once effectively fulfilling and belatedly ennobling his own troubled holy vocation.

CHAPTER 4

THE SURGEON: SURGERY, CHIVALRY, AND SIN
IN THE *PRACTICA* OF JOHN ARDERNE

Introduction

The Middle English version of the Latin *Practica* of the fourteenth-century English surgeon John Arderne opens with the following anecdote: Sir Adam Everingham, a nobleman associated with Henry, earl of Derby (later duke of Lancaster), develops a case of anal fistula, from which he is in a continual state of unbearable pain. He consults doctors and surgeons in Gascony, Bordeaux, Toulouse, and elsewhere, but time and time again is told he is incurable. Giving up hope, Everingham returns home to Tuxford, and, according to Arderne as mediated by his translator, "did of al his kny3tly clothinges and cladde mornyng clothes, in purpose of abydyng dissoluyng, or lesyng, of his body beyng ni3 to hym."[1] Arderne, hearing of Everingham's ailment, "y-sou3t" him out, and, "couenant y-made," heals him within six months. Everingham, newly "hole and sounde," goes on to live another thirty years, while Arderne, for this first successful implementation of his cure for fistula-in-ano, wins "myche honour and louyng þur3 al ynglond" (p. 1).

The point of this story seems, on the surface, little more than a vehicle for the sort of self-advertising common to a profession whose members must assert themselves over competing—and often less qualified—tradesmen, such as barbers, barber-surgeons, and other, independent practitioners. It is also, however, Arderne's first self-conscious linking of surgical activity to a knightly ethos—he is careful to include the chivalric nature of Sir Adam's dress, and contrasts it with the funeral clothing he must change into as his condition worsens. There are contrasting movements at work here. While Everingham's armor, the very sign of his honor and knighthood, is removed, Arderne's honor increases, spreading "þur3 al ynglond." This usurping of his patient's chivalric identity is further evinced by Arderne's having "y-souȝt" Everingham out, a questing action reminiscent of the romance hero. This desire on Arderne's part to share in the knight's signifying economy is, I would suggest, bound up with a deep anxiety over the bodies he routinely encounters, bodies that open, leak, and disintegrate, enacting the most literal sort of fragmentation. Such corporeal horrors would have stood in transgressive opposition to the chivalric aesthetics that Arderne, as a surgeon to such noble clientele, would undoubtedly have absorbed.[2]

The chivalric body is shaped, as Kathleen Kelly has put it, by a "fantasy of intactness,"[3] promulgated in the discursive reiteration of the ideals of muscularity, seamlessness, and virtuous enclosure. What the chivalric body may never be—on peril of nothing less than its status as a signifying subject—is "dissoluyng." Let us linger for a moment upon this curious word. To "dissolve" has, in Middle English, the familiar meaning of "to die," literally to undergo, as the *Middle English Dictionary* (*MED*) puts it, "the separation of body and soul, death."[4] Indeed, the *MED* lists Arderne's lines as an example of such usage. Yet the *MED* also suggests the following meanings: "to break up or dissolve"; "to reduce a solid to a liquid"; "to disintegrate, come to naught"; and other such senses implying the literal dissolution of a substance or being. I believe that Arderne is accessing these more corporeal senses as a subconscious reaction to the raw material of his profession: bodies that dissolve. This chapter will be concerned not only with the horror of the dissolving body, a horror that we will see is inscribed in the language of the *Practica*, but also, to play with the sense somewhat, the "dissolving" of identity. This latter dissolution is in no way separate from that of the body, but is tied inextricably to issues of contour and integrity. The chivalric ethos so present in Arderne's text is, to a large extent, a reaction against this spectacle of the Real, of the body which, through its fissuring and ulcerating, disregards chivalric signification and gives the lie to social coding. Arderne witnesses nothing less than the exposure of the perfectly enclosed chivalric body as, ultimately, a groundless phantasm, and his response, as with the dissolving Adam Everingham, is to privilege, with dogged insistence, the body "hole and sounde."

Critics have recognized for some time now the remarkable similarities between romance imagery and the language of Lacanian psychoanalysis. As Jeffrey Jerome Cohen has noted, Lacan's persistent imaging of identity as a fortress, castle, or armor, corresponds precisely to the enclosed spaces so favored by medieval romance narratives, to the extent that Lacan's account of identity formation "could not have been written had romance been a less culturally formative genre."[5] Such images of fortification are, for Lacan, both a means of description, and objects of psychic archaeology. The function of identity is to enclose the anarchic child-body within an enabling corporeal schema, by which motor discordance might be written over by a controlling physical armor. Yet such culturally received images also occur in dreams, as a means of sustaining this illusion of seamlessness and enclosure.[6] These medieval images of fortresses and armor have persisted as templates of our corporeal mapping, but they also carry with them a transgressive obverse. There are within each of us the submerged memories of a time before coordination, before our orientation within space, which fill us with the lingering anxiety that our fortified contours— the means by which we negotiate our surroundings—are illusory. For Lacan, this anxiety manifests not as castles or other fortified edifices, but as "images of castration, mutilation, dismemberment, dislocation, evisceration, devouring, bursting open of the body," images Lacan groups under the rubric of "the fragmented body."[7] This is the body before social coding, the body prior to the assumption of a corporeal schema (the Imaginary) or subject position (the Symbolic). This is the formless body, the body at the level of the Real.

In various articles and in a monograph, *Of Giants*, Cohen has argued that in the Middle Ages, as now, the prospect of the fragmented body constituted a terrifying threat to identity. This threat manifested in romance narratives as the giant, whose immoderate appetite threatens the hero's dismemberment, his return to "the body before its social containment."[8] This dismembering threat is, in romance, countered by the protagonist's overdetermined heroism, which "organizes the masculine 'body in pieces' into a cultural coherence represented as invulnerable."[9] Thus armed with this phantasmatic invulnerability, the hero performs a symbolic decapitation of the giant, vanquishing the threat of dismemberment that is at once external, and also a condition of his own, internal coherence.

The embodying of this threat of dismemberment is not limited to giants, whose domain is the fantastic, but may also come from more familiar quarters: fellow knights. Kathleen Kelly, in her study of male-male violence in Malory's *Morte Darthur*, focuses on the anxiety that the spectacle of "broken and bloody bodies" holds for the gazing knight.[10] The specular identification between knights is disrupted by the scene of post-combat fragmentation. Bodies that undergo such violence emerge as meaninglessly disordered, and betray the lingering fallibility of the chivalric subject's imagined, idealized lineaments. Without a means of disavowing such a spectacle, "the whole notion of masculine subjectivity will collapse."[11] With the present study, I wish to document a third such threat to phantasmatic identity: the chivalric body under attack from itself. In this way, I mean to close the distance between self and (violent) other, between identity and threat to identity, and show that the most immediate danger to the chivalric subject is the defiant, unpredictable, and unheeding materiality of the body itself, a body that, without warning, can undermine the fantasy of wholeness by means of which the chivalric subject is formed and maintained. Such a project unveils an eerie correspondence between the psychical and the physical, between the twisting and destabilizing of the imaginary borders of identity, and the grisly, bloody deterioration of the flesh itself. No longer monsters of fiction; now, monsters that are "Real."

Fistula-in-Ano and the Dissolving Body

Fistula-in-ano is a condition in which an abscess on the buttocks, left too long unattended, burrows its way through the flesh and, in the worst cases, perforates the rectum. Besides the overwhelming pain, the constant discomfort, the inability to sit or stand for long in a comfortable position, there is the inconvenience of having continual leakage emanate from the fistulate cavities. Although the condition is now exceedingly treatable, Arderne, according to one surgeon and medical historian of the early 1950s, likely saw cases "much more severe than we are accustomed to see to-day."[12] Anal fistula could create one hole on the buttocks, or several; it could involve merely the gluteal region, or encompass the genitalia as well. It is, in effect, a proliferation of anal space, a blurring of the boundaries that delineate corporeal integrity. The borders that mark the division between inside and outside become confused, and the resulting context is one of subversive disorder.

The necessity of the ordered body is promulgated in much medieval philosophy, and most influentially in the work of St. Augustine, who viewed the body as the original paradigm of an ordering principle permeating all Creation. There is a clear opposition within this corporeal hierarchy between positive and negative aesthetic properties:

> And is it not true that in the bodies of animals there are certain members which you could not bear to look at, if you should view them by themselves alone? But the order of nature has designed that because they are needful they shall not be lacking, and because they are uncomely they shall not be prominent. And these ugly members, by keeping their proper places, have provided a better position for the more comely ones what have we ever seen more abject than the deformity of the vanquished one? And yet, by that very deformity was the more perfect beauty of the contest in evidence.[13]

The "deformity" of the ugly members thus plays an essential role in the order of the whole. Their very abjection enables the more "comely" bodily zones to inhabit a privileged signification that would have no meaning if disconnected from this mutually constituting binary. It is when such abject elements exceed their "proper places" that, according to Augustine, they "confuse the whole design."[14] This metaphorical construct does not originate with Augustine in the fourth century, but it occurs throughout the writings of the Classical authorities that precede him. Cicero, in *De natura deorum*, compares the body to an architectural structure, arguing that "just as architects in constructing residences remove from the eyes and noses of their owners the drainage which would inevitably be rather squalid," so too "nature has removed the physical equivalent in our bodies well away from the organs of sense."[15] The excretory organs are thus confined to an abject space where they are not visible, yet, like the sewers of a house, they must exist to protect the schematics by which the lived structure remains socially meaningful. This model applies not only to the literal body, but also to society as metaphorized in medieval literary representations of the "body politic," in which, as Carole Rawcliffe has documented, the lower organs are separated from the upper "as a great landowner might seek to isolate himself from the vulgar herd."[16] Fistula-in-ano must be seen, then, as disordered on several levels: ontological, aesthetic, and social. Needless to say, the psychic implications of engaging with such a condition, let alone suffering its effects, must have been devastating.[17]

Shortly after he cures Sir Adam of this condition, Arderne treats Thomas Brown, who had a total of fifteen abscesses on his buttocks, which were "so vlcerat and putrefied with-in that the quitour and filthe went out ich day als mych as an egg-shel miȝt take" (p. 2). Arderne defines such fistulate conditions in ways that emphasize the regression of the ordered body into a state of viscosity, a movement from delineation to ambiguation. According to Arderne, "a fistule is a depe aposteme, hauyng oonly oon hole somtyme, and ofte-tymes two or þre, and oftymes mo, and bredyng in eche membre of þe body of aposteme or of a wounde yuel y-cured, giffyng out quitour of diuerse colour and of diuerse substaunce" (p. 20). Yet despite this characterization of fistulas as a network of flows and fissures, Arderne, when describing the cases themselves, insists on a language of containment. Brown's pathological liquidity, the emanations that "went out ich day," are crudely spatialized as enough to fill an "egg-shel." The unregulated flow of internal fluids that issue from Brown's body thus is imaged in terms of a containment absent from the spectacle itself, a disavowal of the *non*-containment with which Arderne formally defines the condition. Significantly, the psychoanalyst Didier Anzieu finds that this image is a common expression of corporeal uncertainty. The child first experiences its bodily orifices as a source of anxiety, but gradually develops "the notion of a boundary between the exterior and the interior."[18] As we have seen, however, there remain lingering anxieties that the body is indeed perforated rather than bounded, fears that, according to Anzieu, are "well expressed metaphorically by certain patients who describe themselves as an egg with a broken shell being emptied of its white."[19] The fistula, literally "pipe or tube,"[20] seems an especially potent spectacle of this bodily emptying, and one that Arderne attempts to control through the transformation of the image of the perforated egg into its opposite: an image of containment.

Arderne's desire to contain, then, derives from his specular engagement with bodies that threaten his own sense of coherence. This coherence has been convincingly theorized by Elizabeth Grosz as an "imaginary anatomy," which she defines as an "internalized image or map of the meaning that the body has for the subject, for others in its social world, and for the symbolic order conceived in its generality."[21] Without a unified body image, the subject is indistinguishable from other objects and cannot move or act independently. We live, quite simply, within the limits of our own bodies. Yet these limits are not always fleshly limits but are "extremely fluid and dynamic."[22] Our field of bodily awareness thus expands to include the objects we use as tools. Indeed, Grosz provides an example perfectly germane to the present topic: the surgeon, who "would be unable to operate without the scalpel and medical implements being incorporated into the surgeon's image."[23] Yet if this incorporation of his tools into his body image facilitates Arderne's ability to function as a surgeon, then it also amalgamates him with the very abject bodies upon which he operates.

At many points, Arderne instructs the reader to insert his fingers "in-to þe lure [anus] of þe pacient" (p. 22). Arderne cannot remain uncorrupted throughout this interaction but is drawn into a fusion of "the crossing over of what is touching to what is touched."[24] Touch, because it is the only sense requiring the material coinciding of both parties, has the potential for, in the words of Georges Bataille, "paving the way for a fusion where both are mingled, attaining at length the same degree of dissolution."[25] This "dissolution" cited by Bataille might be defined as the exposure of the subject's spatial autonomy as limited and vulnerable, and this is especially pronounced in the anal conditions that Arderne must treat. The fistula serves to deteriorate flesh and let loose the matter beneath. When situated near or within the anus (the containing organ par excellence), such a condition attests strongly to the fragility of the categories of "inside" and "outside," the supposed division upon which our very subjecthood is founded.

It cannot be forgotten that this was a serious condition that afflicted real people, caused real pain, and terrified patient and doctor alike with the prospects of injury, death, and litigation. Yet there is also an undeniable cultural element at work here. The anus is, of course, already a controversial component of the body, even before this affliction occurs. Arderne inherits not only aspects of his procedure from those who had previously addressed the topic of rectal pathology but also their anxieties. The *Etymologies* of the seventh-century Bishop Isidore of Seville, a text whose influence upon medieval medical theory and terminology cannot be overstated, set an example of squeamishness that later authorities would follow. Like Cicero and Augustine before him, Isidore defines "the posterior parts" as abject, "turned away from the face, lest we be offended by the sight as we empty our bowels."[26] It is this emptying quality, this liquid motion and absence of containment, which, as we shall see, makes the anus so potent a site of anxiety.

This anxiety is passed on to surgical writers. Henri de Mondeville calls the anus a "shameful circle,"[27] while the Catalan surgeon Raimon of Avignon apologizes for pronouncing "such an ugly word."[28] Others associate the anus with filth, as, for example, does an anonymous London surgeon, who, writing in 1392, states that the "ars is þe sercle or þe stynkynge hole out of which hole is cast the draggis, whiche þat ben called dritt."[29] Such a negative view of the anus and excrement is hardly exclusive to surgical or anatomical tracts, but it occurs frequently in medieval poetry as a paradigm of sinfulness. Thus we find, in the Middle English version of Guillaume de Deguileville's dream vision *The Pilgrimage of the Lyfe of the Manhode*, a personification of Lechery who lives in "a verrey dung-hep in a wey-late," and a Gluttony who marks her path with "trases of dunge."[30] It is perhaps because of such sinful associations that Arderne resists naming the anus directly. Instead, he calls it the "lure," which the *MED* defines as the "mouth of a bag." This analogy is not unusual—our anonymous London surgeon concedes that the anus "closiþ like a purs."[31] Yet the fact that other, less extensive treatments of the anus refer to it by its more direct nominations, such as "ers" or "fundement," suggests that Arderne's translator is partaking in an anxious circumlocution.

When confined to its proper place, however, the anus with its excretory function is essential to the perceived bodily order. The anthropologist Mary Douglas, in a statement reminiscent of St. Augustine's views on the ordered body, explains, "Where there is dirt, there is a system."[32] But when this system becomes unbalanced—when "dirt" escapes its confines and spills across boundaries—we respond to the displacement of our ontological dependencies with the appropriate panic and revulsion. Douglas uses the example of the viscous to illustrate the profound effect of experiencing the ambiguation of corporeal borders:

> The viscous is a state half-way between solid and liquid. It is like a cross-section in a process of change. It is unstable, but it does not flow. It is

soft, yielding and compressible. There is no gliding on its surface. Its stickiness is a trap, it clings like a leech; it attacks the boundary between myself
and it. Long columns falling off my fingers suggest my own substance flow-
ing into the pool of stickiness. Plunging into water gives a different impression. I remain a solid, but to touch stickiness is to risk diluting myself into
viscosity.[33]

This "diluting" perfectly characterizes the effects of extreme cases of
fistula-in-ano. To Arderne, the most serious cases are those that most
threaten the integrity of the barriers between inside and outside, liquid and
solid. According to Arderne,

> I haue sene som haue oon hole or many in þe tone buttok, and oon or tuo
> on þe party of þe ȝerde persyng als wele longaon as þe ȝerde. And in þis case,
> as by my demyng, sich pacientes bene vncurable, and þat for fistulyng of þe
> ȝerde. And þat may be knowen, for som-tyme þe sperme goþ oute by þe
> hole of þe ȝerde infistulate, and som-tyme vryne or bothe. (pp. 13–14)

The extent to which a fistula is "vncurable" is tied to the degree to which
the body's form is compromised. This terminal status relates to the loss not
only of the ordered physical body before its fistulate state, but also the loss
of the virtuous identity such a healthy body signifies.

These two levels of the fistula's subverting effects—that of the material
body and of its social signification—are, in this period, inextricably linked.
As Roy Porter explains, "the words 'holiness' and 'healing' stem from a
single root, conveying the idea of wholeness."[34] The fistula, then, not only
fragments the body but, at the same time, corrodes its capacity for signifying a virtuous subject. Indeed, non-virtuous behavior, such as lechery, was
thought to be at the root of a variety of medical complaints. Sickness, in
this period, was understood primarily as the undue gathering of humors in
a particular bodily zone, a state that could be avoided by moderate living
and the avoidance of certain, perilous activities. Hence, surgeons often cite
excessive venality as a cause of fistulate conditions. Our anonymous
London surgeon cautions that the venal patient, "þoruȝ lecherie," engages
in activities that "distempren þe body and meuen þe humouris, whos cours
drawiþ to þe wounde & makiþ it empostime & discrasen."[35] Fistula-in-ano,
then, could be interpreted as a sign of spiritual corruption as well as physical. The fistula is thus "vncurable" in its underminings both of the "whole"
body, and of the "holy" identity.

In the fistulate patients described by Arderne, genitalia, anus, and intervening space coalesce into a nightmarish formlessness, exacerbating an
always precarious sense of bodily integrity. As Douglas notes, these orifices

of the body already "symbolize its especially vulnerable points," since feces, sperm, and other fluids, "by simply issuing forth have traversed the boundary of the body."[36] It is hard to imagine a more transgressive body in Douglas's terms than that of the fistulate patient, whose body is a horrifying realization of the collapsibility that always already inheres in the corporeal structure. One condition that combines these two sites of somatic anxiety—anality and viscosity—is what Arderne calls "bubo within þe lure," which is rectal cancer. Bubo is a state of extreme dissolution, in which the flesh surrounding the anus dissolves, leading eventually to death. Arderne lists the symptoms of bubo as follows: "þai may ete and drynk and go, and somwhat sitte and somwhat slepe; þai be menely hungry and þrifty in mete vnto þe ende; þai may noȝt abstene þam fro þe priuè" (p. 38). In other words, the patient's body ceases to obey rules of containment. Nor does it retain its physiological integrity, for, as Arderne puts it, this condition "fretiþ and wasteþ all þe circumference of it, so þat þe feces of egestiones goþ out continuely vnto þe deth" (p. 37). Death, then, is imaged as the descent into formlessness. Arderne reserves his most emotional language for this condition, admitting that "it may neuer be cured wiþ mannes cure but if it plese god, þat made man of noȝt, for to help wiþ his vnspeakeable vertu" (p. 37). This shift in registers is hardly surprising, given Luke Demaitre's astute observation that it was "in the last phase of medieval pathology, that of description, that authors discussing cancer tended to move from analogy to metaphor, and from dispassionate observation to dramatic representation."[37]

Indeed, this appeal to divine grace is more than merely the commending of a hopeless case to God. Rather, it is a manifestation of the uneasiness Arderne feels in his specular relationship with such profound morbidity. Indeed, death is inscribed into the very terminology by which Arderne figures bubo of the anus. Rectal cancer, he explains, "is callid bubo, for as bubo, i.e. an owle, is a best dwellyng in hideles so þis sikenes lurkeþ wiþin þe lure in þe bikynnyng, but after processe of tyme it vlcerate, & fretyng þe lure goþe out" (p. 37). Arderne's comparison of rectal cancer to an owl is not conceived of autonomously, but is keyed into a tradition that views the owl as a signifier of death and sinfulness. The following passage from an anonymous thirteenth-century Latin bestiary provides us with an example of this negative signification:

> The screech-owl gets its name from the sound of its cry. It is a bird associated with death, burdened with feathers, but bound by a heavy laziness, hovering around graves by day and night, and living in caves. The screech-owl is an image of all those who live in the darkness of sin and flee the light of justice. It is known as a loathsome bird because its roost is filthy from its

droppings, just as the sinner brings all who dwell with him into disrepute through the example of his dishonourable behavior. It is burdened with feathers to signify an excess of flesh and levity of spirit, always bound by a heavy laziness, the same laziness which binds sinners who are inert and idle when it comes to doing good. It lives by day and night in graveyards, just like sinners who delight in their sin, which is the stench of human flesh.[38]

The owl is "associated with death" not only literally, as a creature preferring the morbid surroundings of graveyards, but also psychically. The owl has no life outside the realm of the abject, for its contours betray its ambiguous form and absence of containment. "Burdened with feathers," and layered with "an excess of flesh," the owl is an appropriate specter of formlessness with which to oppose the once "hole and sounde" forms of those knightly patients whose identities have been compromised by these ambiguating conditions. Indeed, so pervasive was the link between death and rectal pathology that some authorities, such as the thirteenth-century Italian surgeon Theodoric Borgognoni, apply to anal fistulas the characteristic of postmortem rotting of the flesh, insisting that "a worm can issue from them."[39] For the patient afflicted with anal fistula, especially the knightly patient, the prospect of death is twofold, like that death which the owl so frightfully embodies. Indeed, the patient's death is not merely that which potentially awaits him at the denouement of that foreboding temporal construction "vnto þe deth," but also death at the levels of both the Symbolic and the Imaginary. A knight so afflicted cannot ride on horseback, cannot bear arms, and, in short, may not engage in any of the identity practices that afford him so privileged a position within the Symbolic. Nor can the body, thus ravaged and assaulted, accommodate any longer the imaginary contours that once bound it so precariously to the idealized template of chivalric identification. All at once, the illusion of the chivalric body is exposed.

Treatment and Containment

The medieval treatment of fistula-in-ano derives ultimately from Latin translations of Arabic sources, which in turn are based upon Greco-Roman authorities. Generally, anal fistulas in specific are dealt with within larger sections concerning fistulas in general or are confined to a single chapter. Arderne's focus on the condition is anomalous, prompting Peter Murray Jones to write, "We should be surprised to find such an extensive treatment of any surgical specialty in the scholastic authors, above all not for such an unglamorous subject as fistula-in-ano."[40] The twelfth-century Arabic authority Albucasis is thought to be the most likely source for Western approaches to fistula-in-ano. In the case of perforating fistulas, Albucasis, like many subsequent authorities, considers intervention to be generally futile. He does give instructions for cautery, cutting, and lancing but, anxious of the last two, recommends cauterization as the least injurious approach.[41] He also gives instructions for ligature—the tying of a thread through the fistulate cavity and out through the rectum—as a means of slowly slicing the intervening flesh without the trauma of direct incision. His works are first quoted by Theodoric Borgognoni in the thirteenth century, who modifies them by showing how ligature can be used to secure the flesh for incision, and not just for its laborious, sawing effect.[42] Yet despite these resources for dealing with the condition, many near contemporaries of Arderne, including Henri de Mondeville and Lanfranco, advise against any active surgical intervention.

Hence, when Arderne comes to devise his treatment, and to witness its relative success, he can hardly be blamed for his self-congratulatory tone: "And this I sey that I know noȝt in al my tyme, ne hard not in al my tyme, of any man, nouþer in yngland ne in partieȝ biȝond þe see, that kouthe cure fistula in ano" (p. 3). He does not simply overcome surgical apprehension and employ available yet neglected knowledge; he defines himself by his investments in anal conditions. Indeed, he proudly proclaims his invention of new instruments for the purpose.[43] Most authorities before him, such as Albucasis, de Mondeville, and Lanfranco, warn the reader about the dangers of an accidental cut to the sphincter; Arderne invented the *coclear*, a spoon-like implement that, when placed against the rectal wall, shields the excretory tract from accidental perforation when the surgeon cuts the fistulate passage. This instrument "shal defende þe lure þat it be noȝt hurt. . .wiþ þe poynt of þe rasour or of þe launcette" (p. 24). That he describes this shielding function in terms of a defensive armament is not surprising, given that it is the illusion of the body as armor that is at stake.

It is telling that Arderne would devise an instrument specifically for this purpose, he who is so unusual in recommending cutting above all other options. Incision is merciful compared to ligature, which can take days, even weeks, to work its way through the flesh; yet it was approached with trepidation by medieval surgeons, in part because of ecclesiastical injunctions against the higher orders shedding blood,[44] but also because, as Marie Pouchelle points out, "penetrating the body—the microcosm—meant interfering in a transcendent interplay of forces."[45] Arderne's language attests to this trepidation. The surgeon, he states, should "*boldly* kutte the flesshe" (p. 24). He repeats this adverbial qualification several times throughout the treatise, displaying an awareness of the transgression involved in duplicating, with the razor, the destructive and disordering effects of the fistula itself. Following the incision, hemorrhage is stanched using a series of sponges or with a "lynnen girdel" (p. 25), and Arderne is peculiar as well in giving such detailed instructions for coping with this problem. His innovations are concentrated upon maintaining the integrity of the body, his instruments and instructions ensuring that internal matter does not traverse its conventional boundaries. Arderne, even more than most surgeons of his day, is obsessed that the limits of the body remain intact.

In this role of containment, Arderne acts as a keeper of the body, a self-appointed arbiter of the socially corporeally permissible. Indeed, he assumes in post-operative care the role of a parental authority, instructing the patient to abstain from defecating so that the medicated gauze he must wear remains attached to the affected area. The patient, of course, must eventually violate these instructions, "ʒitte he be amonysched to abstine" (p. 26). Julia Kristeva, in her psychoanalytic reworking of Mary Douglas, posits such fecal regulation as an originary factor in the subject's orientation within the Symbolic, arguing that "maternal authority is experienced first and above all, after the first essentially oral frustrations, as sphincteral training."[46] According to Kristeva, it is through this maternal admonishment that we first experience language in all its limiting and formative power. The smell and appearance of excrement become the template not merely for our notion of revulsion, but also for our understanding of what constitutes subject and object, inside and outside. It is telling, therefore, that Arderne often describes fistula-in-ano in terms of its excremental qualities, as issuing matter "wiþ gret hete and stynk" (p. 41)—a common enough observation in medieval surgical literature. Almost all conditions, including fistula-in-ano, were thought to be caused by the disproportionate gathering, stagnating, and, subsequently, corrupting, of the body's humoral fluids. These humors, in their corrupted state, are often characterized by surgeons and physicians alike as having a malodorous smell, as when Lanfranco emphatically describes an afflicted patient as "stynkynge, and þat riʒt foul stynkyng."[47] It is difficult to say whether such a description is fully the result of sensory observation, or is a sub- or self-conscious conformity on the surgeon's part to established physiological theory regarding the humors. As John Trevisa explains, "in a body wiþ euel odour ben corrump humours, for þe kynde qualitees þerof ben oute passed."[48] In his *Canon of Medicine*, Avicenna describes such "corrump humours" as having a "foul acid smell which even the flies shun."[49]

The importance of olfactory descriptions of ulcerate wounds to the present discussion goes beyond the (admittedly simple) task of itemizing fistula-in-ano's repulsive qualities. That surgeons describe such wounds as malodorous is significant in ways that are far more psychically fraught. Smell, in the Middle Ages, was thought to contain the essence of the thing perceived. To smell a thing is to absorb it on a material level. Thomas Norton, an alchemist of the fifteenth century, provides a typical definition of "stynche" as the "res-olued fumosite" of something rotting, the "corrupcion of the selfe sub-stance."[50] As Trevisa points out, such "stynkynge þinges" are by no means passive or benign, but "bredeþ sodeynliche corrupcion in hole men."[51] The limits of the body thus are even more permeable, more open to attack, than they would first appear. It is because of this conception of smell as malign that much of western Europe, made wary by the widespread destruction caused by the Black Death, imposed strict regulations upon all practices that could incur corrupt odors, such as sewage disposal, street cleaning, and the keeping and discarding of foodstuffs.[52] Smells, then, posed a very real threat to the body "hole and sounde." Arderne's containing treatments are an attack not only upon the visible leakage that escapes the confines of the body, but also upon the airborne corruption that issues forth from within its borders. The matter that spews from the fistulate body is thus beyond spatialization, beyond dimensionalization, but emanates pervasively, in the most transgres-sive mode of formlessness.

By regulating such matter, Arderne functions in a similar way to Kristeva's maternal authority, who, in her regulating of the child's defeca-tory output, effects the originary "mapping of the self's clean and proper body."[53] In demanding that the recovering patient apply gauzes to his wounds and suppress defecation, he reinstates the enclosed body by forcing the patient to undertake the performative containment of its openings. Despite the practical necessity of "closing" the patient, we might speculate that Arderne's enclosing methodology has as much to do with his own body as that of his patient's. As a surgeon whose clientele was culled largely from a knightly milieu, he lived in a world of masculine specularity, in which chivalric identities were assumed in a fluctuating cycle of circula-tion, activation, and imitation. For him to gaze daily upon his patients and their (to return to Kelly's phrase) "broken and bloodied bodies," was to engage in specular alignment with the distorted and collapsed proofs of the impossibility of the perfectly sealed chivalric body. It is to realize, in short, the instability upon which all bodies, including his own, are founded.

Does Arderne effect these innovations to protect himself from the hor-ror of the dissolving subject, or is it his own libidinal fascination that he wishes, on some level, to contain? Georges Bataille draws our attention to the potential for the dissolving body to evoke not just horrific, but erotic sensations. He defines the erotic as the achievement of a "degree of dissolution," a breaking down of the psychically enforced borders that divide the body from its surrounding space.[54] For Bataille, such dissolution functions as a way of compromising with the constraints of the lived body. There are, Bataille suggests, "unmistakable links between excreta, decay, and sexuality";[55] each give subjects that experience them access to a mode of radical continuity with that beyond their bodies. To Mary Douglas, such dissolution is an occasion for profound unease, but to Bataille, it is a means of surmounting the crippling anxieties that always accompany the self-confinement of the subject to a lived (and limited) body. Violence, intercourse, defecation, all of these can be used as performative modes with which to disengage ourselves, however briefly, from the act of regarding our bodies as bounded and autonomous. Our access to such liberation is limited by our training, received in childhood, to feel nausea at anything linked to excrement, to decay, and, in turn, to death. As Bataille argues in Ciceronian fashion, "The sexual channels are the body's sewers; we think of them as shameful and connect the anal orifice with them."[56] Eroticism is therefore seldom experienced directly but is most often accessed through ritual, through spectatorship, through witnessing social and physical boundaries being violated under more or less official conditions.

For Bataille, such spectatorial occasions are usually sacrificial. Sacrificial occasions function as a means of circumventing the traumatic effects of collapsing our own corporeal borders, an action that would require self-mutilation. By sanctioning the spectacle of another's dissolution, we share in that catharsis. Such occasions, argues Bataille, induce a "revelation of continuity through the death of a discontinuous being to those who watch it as a solemn rite."[57] Medieval surgery has a similarly performative aspect. It can be argued that nowhere in medieval society was there per-mitted as much extended tactile interaction with the body, as much pur-poseful exceeding of bodily limits, as in the surgical situation. Not even the marriage bed permitted such licentious roving across the corporeal terrain. Arderne insists upon a series of ritualized actions before his incisions can begin. He instructs the reader to have "þe pacient ledde to a place made redy Where þe lech shal do mynystryng of a cure," then to give a practiced speech urging the patient to cooperate in the procedure (p. 23). Throughout, the surgery may be witnessed by fellows of the surgeon, a spectatorial component that adds greatly to surgery's sense of ritual.

When placed in the broader context of a chivalric society, however, surgery must be seen as an engagement with bodies that are themselves transgressive and utterly discomfiting. Indeed, surgery and chivalry share a variety of characteristics, both (and at once) discursive and historical. Although the potential for Arderne's work to invoke an erotic release from the anxieties of maintaining a chivalric identity is interesting to consider, the evidence points far more to a shared, somatic horror on the parts of both surgical and chivalric writers. The following section will examine the ethos of violence shared between these two sorts of texts and their consid-erable overlap as generic "types."

The Sword and the Scalpel

Arderne seems to have discovered the interchangeability of signification that bound the knight and the surgeon to each other as subjects founded upon violence. As professionals whose livelihood depended upon their manual prowess, both knights and surgeons came to be identified, like craftsmen, by their tools. The surgeon's instruments performed much the same functions as the knight's weapons: cutting, piercing, and tearing human flesh. In his *Chirurgia magna*, the fourteenth-century French surgeon Guy de Chauliac, who we have encountered many times, defines one group of indispensable surgical instruments as "yren instrumentis," of which "some beeþ to kutte wiþ, as scheres, rasoures and launcetes."[58] In descriptions of these tools, we often find overlap between the knightly and the surgical. Henri de Mondeville, for one, describes the *crepanum*, a surgical instrument used for incision, as "a blad scherynge on boþe sidis *as a swerd*, þat if a man turne þe shaft bitwixe hise hondis, it perseþ þe brayn-panne."[59] This shared terminology also occurs in the other direction, such as in *Sir Gawain and the Green Knight*, where the Green Knight's deadly (and surgically precise) axe is described as "wel schapen to schere as scharp rasores."[60] In each case, the intention is to illustrate the destructive potential of the described object, a tacit acknowledgment of their shared economy of violence.

De Mondeville, in the same passage where he compares the crepanum to a sword, describes another surgical tool as "sich an instrument as carpenteris maken." This analogy is not surprising, given that surgery was in this period associated with craft, both etymologically and professionally. Isidore of Seville's popular construction—that the word "surgery" is a compound of the Greek words *cyros* (hand) and *agia* (action)—retained its appeal throughout the later Middle Ages, and especially so in England, where surgery was controlled by guilds long after it had begun to be taught scholastically on the Continent.[61] In this practical field, it is experience that is the best teacher, and this is perhaps the foremost distinction between surgeons and their more conventionally scholastic counterparts, the physicians. Arderne is on many occasions emphatic that in surgery, one cannot rely on books alone:

> For al þings þat ow to be done about sich werk may noȝt be expressed in letterȝ, and þerfor it byhoueþ a crafty [lech] to be wise and slyȝe wele ymagynyng subtile þings, þat in þose þings þat perteneþ to þe perfitenes of þis werk and aboue al þings þat he has lerned in þis boke he may availe hym þurȝ benefice of his ovne witte. (p. 23)

These two qualities—the manual and the experiential—are also essential to the man at arms. The *Book of Fayttes of Armes*, a Caxtonian translation of

Christine de Pizan's guide to chivalry, insists that the knight should, "by longe experyence," be able to perform his duties "as a naturel crafte or mestier."[62] Indeed, craftsmen are regarded by Pizan as naturally inclined toward the art of fighting, since each involves the direct exertion of force upon a body or object. Christine de Pizan is clear on the point that, if a captain is short of men and needs must recruit,

> he ought singulerly to chese theym that can som craftes / as bochers that are woned to shede bloode & to smyte with axes / carpenters smythes and all other exersyce theyre bodyes in trauaill and in werkes that be doon by might of mannys hand. . .[63]

The compatibility of carpentry, and other manual crafts, with the act of fighting, is evinced not only by such instructions from chivalric treatises, but also by fictional representations of those instructions in action. In the Arthurian romance *Of Arthour and of Merlin*, for example, Arthur and his knights, in combat with the pagans, "hewen on wiþ gret powers / On schides so doþ þis carpenters."[64] Surgeons themselves often describe their particular type of "hewing" as resembling that of craftsmen, such as when Raimon of Avignon instructs the surgeon sewing a severed jugular vein to "be like an artisan."[65] Because the art of surgery, like knighthood, was associated with tasks that required "the might of mannes hand," surgeons were expected to have the same physical attributes of muscularity and good proportion as their knightly counterparts. Henri de Mondeville, to cite just one example, insists that the surgeon have "membris stronge, þat he be my3ti to do alle oþere manere operaciouns þat him owiþ to do."[66]

Yet Arderne, at the same time, speaks of strength largely in spiritual terms, as if attempting to lift his discourse above this bodily emphasis. Almost from the outset, he declares that "he, forsoþe, þat is wayke of herte is no3t in way of curacion" (p. 7). He is harsh to weak men, whom he calls "feble men," because "al þing3 bene hard to a waik hert man," but to "a strong hert man, forsoþ, is noþing grete" (p. 64). This privileging of spiritual over physical strength is a strategy that Arderne borrows from chivalric writings to disavow the corporeal emphasis of his profession. This strategy is most pronounced in Ramon Lull's *Order of Chivalry*, in which Ramon Lull frequently de-emphasizes the aspect of the physical, so central to his treatise, by demanding of the knight that "in his herte he haue strengthe," rather than in "the nature of the body."[67] This is necessary, reasons Lull, because

> yf chyualrye were more stronge of body / than in strengthe and courage / ordre of Chyualrye shold more accorde to the body than to the soule And yf it were so the body shold be more noble than the soule / but that is openly fals.[68]

In this fashion, chivalric writers frequently deny the centrality of the body to their discourses. By consistently privileging the heart over the body, Arderne seems to share with chivalry this strategy for transcending the overtly corporeal nature of his own treatise.

Yet there is also a medical basis for this "weakness of the heart." The weakhearted man is not always so by choice, but the reason lies in the fact that he is often burdened with that inadequacy as a result of his physiological complexion. Avicenna, in a tract on cardiac pathology, defines weakness of heart as the result of humoral determinants, of "coldness of blood and its scarcity and thinness."[69] This deficiency of vital heat "slackens the motive powers" and impels those it afflicts to flee objects of fear rather than confront them.[70] Surgery and chivalry each present their practitioners with gory bodies, objects of fear par excellence, and therefore require individuals of an altogether different humoral makeup. In this way, the language of strong-heartedness provides a correspondingly deterministic apposite to the chivalric myth of the origin of knighthood, which Lull depicted so influentially as God's selection of the "most stronge" man that occurs in every thousand.[71] Arderne, who displays a knowledge of scholastic medicine throughout his *Practica*, likely understood the "waik hert" not only as a metaphor for cowardice, but also as a physiological condition that problematized the treatment of certain individuals, and excluded others from becoming surgeons. Nor is the application to chivalry as well as surgery lost on Arderne, who will occasionally use martial metaphors to describe surgical practice. For example, he warns against allowing excessive loss of blood, a naturally curative substance, by stating that "if þe frende be destroyed þe enemy waxeþ miȝty" (p. 60). It is far from disjunctive for him to borrow from chivalric discourses—the two professions share a similar methodology: each works directly, and with extraordinary violence, upon the body.

This violence integral to both the knight and the surgeon served to identify each as potential threats, each as potent an adversary to the body "hole and sounde" as were the lawlessness and sickness which, respectively, it was their jobs to defeat. Geoffroi de Charny seizes on this point when he condemns those knights who would "wage war without good reason, who seize other people without prior warning and without good cause rob and steal from them, wound and kill them."[72] The *Lanterne*-author also harshly rebukes those knights who do not focus their violence upon the lawless, but instead engage in "fiȝtynge euer anoon."[73] This anxiety, although it may seem hyperbolic, is understandable given the normalizing treatment afforded violent dismemberment in chivalric treatises. The following is an especially horrific example from *Knyghthode and Bataile*, in which the author joyfully advocates the most merciless of fighting strategies:

> Empeche his hed, his face, have at his gorge,
> Bere at the breste, or s[e]rue him on the side
> With myghti knightly poort, eue as Seynt George,
> Lepe o thi foo, loke if he dar abide;
> Wil he nat fle, wounde him; mak woundis wide,
> Hew of his honde, his legge, his thegh, his armys;
> It is the Turk: though he be sleyn, noon harm is.[74]

Dismemberment, the disordering of limbs and the dismantling of limits, is presented here as a noble mode of combat, and is endorsed, joltingly, through no less a national and chivalric icon than St. George. Just a few lines later, the reader is told to eschew crude swings for pointed jabs, or *foynes*, because the most damage may be done through the breaching of the entrails, which "ar couert in steel & bonys" (l. 379). The enclosing armor that is so integral to knightly identity is here conflated with the body itself—"steel & bonys" form the outer shell that not only protects the knight but defines his body's contours. There is no spatial distinction made here between the organic and the constructed; the two are conflated in a way that emphasizes their interdependence in the maintenance of chivalric identity. At the same time as the knight pierces these layers in another, he also compromises the extent to which his own illusion of an armored form may be psychically sustained. Although the author attempts to insert a reassuring distance between the knight and his opponent through the othering nomination "Turk," the emphasis here is on the penetration of innards, bones, and sinews, an engagement with the Real. Such binaristic encoding unravels drastically when we consider that the phrase "woundis wide," for the damage that the knight is charged with inflicting upon the unholy body of the Saracen, also commonly refers to those wounds inflicted upon the paradigmatically sacred body of Jesus Christ.[75] Lurking beneath the clearly distinguished nominations "Turk" and "Christian," then, lies a dangerous instability, and the ever-present potential for both body and its signification to fragment uncontrollably.

The fearfulness that attended the errant knight is also evident in social reactions to surgery as a growing profession. The potential for the surgical art to reveal the bone and gristle obscured in corporeal formation was combated, appropriately, on the level of the visual. London barbers were, in 1307, instructed by the mayor not to leave bowls of blood in shop windows where they could disturb passersby, while in Paris barbers were told to dispose quickly of such grisly material.[76] Surgeons, coming to recognize this social apprehension that accompanied their development as a profession, sought to police their own ranks. In 1375, the Guild of Barbers drew up an ordinance appointing two of its members to "oversee the tools of all the said art that they be good and fitting for the use of the people to avoid the peril which might happen."[77] The 1423 Charter of the short-lived Conjoint College of Physicians and Surgeons in London expresses a similar anxiety over practitioners performing cures from "whiche may folowe Dethe or mayme."[78] Before long, this fear of a disordering violence in surgery extended beyond the operating room, and into the surgical community itself, as we see from regulations drafted by the Government of the Guild of Surgeons in 1435 prohibiting any of the fellowship to "drawe ony wepene in violence or unlawfulli manace ony persoone of the seid crafte."[79] Like the knight's, the surgeon's identity was bound up with violence. Trained to protect, the knight is also trained to kill. Trained to heal, the surgeon is also taught to cut, to burn, and to dismember.

Surgical and chivalric treatises, because they share an ethos of violence, also come to share an anxious self-regulation, an insistence upon their own bodies as positively distinct from those collapsed bodies with which they are trained to engage. The traumatic effects of witnessing dismemberment are well attested to in chivalric treatises. To be a knight is to acclimatize oneself through a normalizing regimen to the spectacle of the Real, as the following passage from *Knyghthode and Bataile* makes clear:

> Thus hardy hem; for whos is vnexpert
> Of werre, and woundis seeth, and summe slayn,
> He weneth euery strok go to his hert,
> And wiste he how, he wolde fle ful fayn.
> But and he fle, retourne him fast agayn.
> Thus with seueritee and good vsage
> Ther wil revive in theim a fyne corage.
>
> (ll. 1664–70)

This somatic anxiety that haunts the chivalric subject is met by the disavowing strategy of an overdetermined bodily wholeness. The knight must not identify with those splattered bodies, but he must retain the fantasy of intactness that distinguishes his own contours from those of the bloodied casualties. The incomplete or poorly shaped body is thus abjected from the chivalric signifying economy. Chivalric voices attest harshly to this abjectifying principle, most notably Ramon Lull, who states that a man "ouer grete or ouer fatte," "lame of ony membre," or "that hath ony other euyl disposycion in his body," is not "dygne ne worthy to be receiued in to thordre of chyualrye."[80] In this fashion, Lull and others repeatedly emphasize the chivalric body as one of unerring proportion, as the body "hole and sounde." Such persistent reiteration of the ideal chivalric body allows the knight to imagine his own lineaments as formed outside of discourse, as mandated by a knightly *ordre* (order) that is transcendent and autonomous, rather than imposed through what Judith Butler has called "a process of materialization that stabilizes over time to produce the effect of boundary, fixity, and surface we call matter."[81] The phantasmatic body thus acts preemptively, providing in advance a psychical opposition to the knight's specular engagement with the "woundis" of the dead and injured forms that surround him. Such monstrous wounds belie the fantasy of an impenetrable bodily armor, yet, in the same instance as they are seen by the knight, they are (it is hoped) written over by the unremitting internalization of a body image that appears seamless and contained. It is no wonder that surgical writers, who are almost always practitioners as well, and thus similarly inured to the spectacle of fragmented bodies, also insist upon the physical intactness of their fellows. Among other, more intellectual qualifications, Guy de Chauliac would have the surgeon be "well-þewed," a quality not only necessary for restraining struggling patients during an operation but also an anxious invocation of the virtuous chivalric form.[82]

This ideal body image of the complete and sealed knight is promulgated not only discursively but performatively as well. The realities of the knightly body are disavowed through a set of identity practices emphasizing the sleek contours of an enclosing armor. The author of *Knyghthode and Bataile* recommends an almost prosthetic relationship of the knight to his armor, prescribing an exercise in which the knight must "se that euery peece herneys be sure," and, thus enclosed, "Go quyckly in, and quyk out of the gere" (l. 491). So bound should the body of the knight be to the contours of his armor that even the prostrate form of the knight in repose should conform to this "entatched" ideal. We need look no further than *Sir Gawain and the Green Knight* to find a knight who, in pursuit of the chivalric ideal, "sleped in his yrnes" (l. 729). Also, to quote a more overtly parodic example, the beloved lady of *The Squire of Low Degree* lists for her less-than-prestigious suitor a number of knightly conventions with which to "gette your name," concluding with the requirement that "in your armure must ye lie."[83] Both these romances occur late in the development of the genre and present extremely self-aware, almost comical depictions of an unsustainable knightly identity. Such examples therefore serve to illustrate the enduring power of the image of the knight bonded to his armor, an image I would suggest is more than a fictive conceit, it is also a literary representation of a potent identificatory practice.

In chivalric treatises, the desire for containment is evinced most powerfully in the convention of listing each piece of armor with its corresponding significance. In many cases, armor acts as a microcosmic fortress, those military enclosures that, insists *Knyghthode and Bataile*, must "stonde an infallibil thing for euer" (l. 2267). Such a description returns us to Cohen's assertion of the indebtedness of Lacanian theories of identity formation to the language of chivalry. Knightly identity is predicated upon the illusion of the body as "infallibil." Ramon Lull, when itemizing pieces of the armor of a knight, argues that the hauberk "sygnefyeth a castel & fortresse ageynst vyces & deffaultes"; this formulation depends upon an aesthetics of enclosure; just as "a castel and fortresse ben closed al aboute," so too "an hauberke is ferme & cloos on al partes."[84] The author of the Wyclifite treatise *Lanterne of Liȝt* restates the notion of an "harburioune of riȝtwisenesse," but adds an item not listed by Lull: a "girdil of chastite."[85] Both hauberk and girdle not only symbolize the good knight's immunity to sin but also suggest the degree to which chivalry is obsessed with the firmness and seamlessness of its bodies. This desire to enclose the body is juxtaposed, problematically, with the teleology of combat, which we have already seen illustrated so gorily as the piercing and opening of the corporeal structure.

Where chivalry invokes such articles of dress to symbolize (and enforce) its fantasy of bodily intactness, surgical writings often incorporate sartorial imagery in ways that evince the very instability of that idealized form. Knights, for all their violent rhetoric, may have experienced tournaments or wars intermittently, or for short periods of time. The surgeon, who is professionally bound to witness the dissolution of the ulcerated body, seems unable to sustain such a fantasy of wholeness. This anxiety is especially pronounced in descriptions of Arderne's specialty, fistula-in-ano. In a Middle English version of the surgery of the thirteenth-century Montpellier surgeon William of Congeinna, the "girdil of chastite," whose definition requires that it remain intact, gives way to a corrosive converse: "þe fretyng girtel"[86] that "fretiþ aboute þe place þat he sit on."[87] For Arderne, as well, the girdle is not an enclosing armor but an apparatus that takes the body formless and dissolving as the condition of its existence. He prescribes for the post-operative staunching of fluids a "wolnen girdel or a lynnen" (p. 25), whose fate is to be removed when it has become too dense with corpuscular and fecal matter to maintain its circumscribing hold. Where in chivalry armor is used to circumscribe the contours of the complete body, here it denotes the fretting and disintegrating of those previously intact lineaments.

These abject elements so commonly witnessed by the surgeon comprise the main matter of much romance narrative, where the opening and piercing of bodies are enacted with a stultifying frequency. Romance authors, however, have recourse to a plethora of disavowing fictions with which to distance the perfect bodies they privilege from the grisly specters with which those bodies become enmeshed. The monster of romance, for example, may be one means to externalize the lingering threat of exposure that resides within each chivalric body. Jeffrey Jerome Cohen points out that this fantastic embodiment most often takes the form of the giant, who is often "an allegory for gluttony," and "embodies appetite of all kinds."[88] This representation of the abject as devouring applies equally to surgical discourses. Surgeons find their own form of disavowal in representing the wounds that they encounter as similarly monstrous. Just as giants are often characterized by a "feral mouth that devours,"[89] and are nullified by the romance hero in a decapitation that affirms his own coherence, so too are the wounds treated by surgeons often figured in terms of a similarly voracious orality.

Theodoric, Arderne's foremost influence in the development of his surgical method, describes fistulate wounds as having "thick *lips* on the ulcer and hard," adding that "sometimes it closes, and sometimes it opens."[90] Our anonymous London surgeon reveals that a cancerous wound may be known by its "hauynge greete *lippis* sumdeel ouerturned and vprerid, cauernous or hollowʒ, hard, knoti, pale and blak."[91] Arderne himself tells us that, in the case of one patient, he "perceyued þat þe place was disposed to þe fistule, for it had ane hole or a *mouþe* and a depe wonde" (p. 48). The fistula not only resembles a mouth, but, like Cohen's romance monster, possesses a "gross, ingestive corporeality."[92] To illustrate this point, Arderne describes one of his patients as so ravished by this condition that "þe lure was vtterly *gnawen* away" (p. 39). The wound, then, is itself a monster. Yet whereas the romance monster is at once destructive and affirming, both a threat to, and condition of, the knight's own internal coherence, the fistula does not allow for such a tidy disavowal. Its landscape is not the anonymous forest of romance, but the flesh itself. This monster cannot be relegated to a fictive outside, nor contained within narrative space, but claws its way up from within subjectivity. Faced with such an enemy, it is no wonder that Arderne clings to this ideal of the chivalric body, to the illusion of the "hole and sounde."

Indeed, Arderne can be seen to be maneuvring through the same sort of ambiguous landscape as the knight of romance. Bakhtin has written influentially of the romance landscape as a terrain through which

> the hero moves from country to country, comes into contact with various masters, crosses various seas—but everywhere the world is one, it is filled with the same concept of glory, heroic deed and disgrace; throughout this world the hero is able to bring glory on himself and on others; everywhere the same names resound and are glorious.[93]

This conflation of space and time into an ambiguous oneness is similar to Arderne's anomalous concentration upon the anus. He eschews the head-to-toe organization that is traditional in scholastic surgical writings, and instead presents a disunified, often rambling treatise focusing on the area that surrounds the anus. The patient's body is not broken down, as was customary, into components but, like Bakhtin's romance landscape, is a homogenized surface replete with monsters and dangerous crossings. Like the hero of romance, the goal of the surgeon is to achieve honor and lasting fame. This is especially pronounced for Arderne, for whom no university education or affiliation can be proven. His professional life, it would seem, was tied to secular society. He, more than his scholastic counterparts, positions himself as competitive, stating scornfully that instead of attempting to treat fistula-in-ano, his contemporaries "kest it vtterly byhinde þair bak" (p. 3). Needless to say, the punning diction of this sentence suggests that Arderne's first thought was to describe an anatomical act of an altogether more awkward nature.

When Arderne first began to defeat these monsters of the body, the "duke of lancastre and many othir gentiles wondred ther-of" (p. 1). It would seem that, in many ways, he is partaking of the same economy of honor as was expected of the knight. His desire to make known the uniqueness of his successes conforms strongly to the interplay, integral to the formation of chivalric identity, between knightly performance and public validation. Geoffroi de Charny describes this potent interplay in terms stunningly similar to recent, Lacanian-inspired accounts of gender construction, such as those of Judith Butler and Elizabeth Grosz. Such accounts work to contravene the essentializing mandate of Western approaches to the body, approaches that seek to define gender characteristics as innate and prediscursive. The body is the result of countless and fluctuating internalizations of cultural norms, and thus it is never autonomous or independent of the discourses of its society. As Grosz puts it, "The 'natural' body, insofar as there is one, is continually augmented by the products of history and culture, which it readily incorporates into its own intimate space."[94]

In de Charny's *The Book of Chivalry*, there is a similar appreciation of the role specularity and mimesis play in the formation of the subject. The very real effects of discourse upon the material bodies that absorb it are attested to in the following passage, which uses the example of the maturation of a boy into knighthood to illustrate the mimetic nature of chivalry:

> It is embodied in those who, from their own nature and instinct, as soon as they begin to reach the age of understanding, like to hear and listen to men of prowess talk of military deeds, and to see men-at-arms with their weapons and armour and enjoy looking at fine mounts and chargers; and as they increase in years, so they increase in prowess and in skill in the art of arms in

peace and war; and as they reach adulthood, the desire in their hearts grows ever to ride horses and to bear arms. And they themselves, through their great zeal and determination, learn the true way to practise the military arts, until they, on every occasion, know how to strive toward the most honourable course of action, whether in relation to deeds of arms or in relation to other forms of behavior appropriate to their rank.[95]

The noble child, at the supposed genesis of his cognitive awareness, absorbs the images of the bodies around him, bodies defined as chivalric by their weaponry, horse, and armor. These keen edges, muscled beasts, and plated contours thus become the template of his own self-perception. Just as, for Butler, the subject's imagined body "stabilizes over time," so too does Charny's maturing knight "increase in prowess." As each stage is reached, still more is required, since "the more these men see and themselves perform brave deeds, the more it seems to them, because of the high standards their natural nobility demands of them, that they have done nothing."[96] Once this valor is achieved, the knight can expect to display an outward identity as if it were a "garment" that is "embroidered and richly worked with the qualities" of the chivalric knight.[97] There is, implicit in this construction of a "garmented" knight, the specter of his naked opposite, a valuative dichotomy corresponding strongly to the distinction, made previously, between the intact and dissolving girdles.[98] Once again, the successful assumption of identity is linked to the image of the bounded physical self.

Those who do not conform to this identificatory regime become abjected, and signify little in the world that de Charny depicts. Such casualties of signification are necessary, argues Butler, to ensure that "the domain of the subject will circumscribe its own autonomy and life."[99] De Charny illustrates this interdependence between the subject and the abject through the example of a courtly dinner. Two women wait for their respective suitors to enter the hall, one of whom is a knight "celebrated by all manner of people," the other "a miserable wretch" who, "for no good reason, is unwilling to bear arms."[100] According to de Charny, it is a matter of course that the lady with the famous lover will be more pleased, while she whose lover cannot signify as a knight is shamed. De Charny communicates to us the contrasting positions these two bodies occupy on the scale of social significance by describing their different receptions at hall. While the knight is "honoured, saluted, and celebrated," the other "remains hidden behind everyone else." By not enacting the identification practices germane to knightly identity, this latter suitor is abjected into a domain where he has no "autonomy and life," but is socially invisible, even, we might say, symbolically dead. This failure to engage in the performative repetition of the chivalric norms he has absorbed causes him, as Ramon Lull remarks pointedly of the lawless knight, to "deffeate a knyght in hym self."[101]

That Arderne and de Charny are each concerned with receiving the proper public validation reflects the extent to which some surgeons, by the later Middle Ages, had access to chivalric society. According to the *Liber niger* of the Household of Edward IV, the surgeon was entitled to a "knyʒtes lyuery," and, when sick, could procure "squyers for the body."[102] Given the immense influence of chivalric discourses upon aristocratic society, the prominence of the surgeon at court meant an inevitable conformity of surgical to knightly discourse.[103] This is especially evident in the issue of conduct. Both chivalric and surgical treatises provide, in what might be considered subgenres of their respective types, lists of the qualities possessed by their ideal representatives. Often, both types of treatise match each other point for point in this regard. Arderne requires of the surgeon that, among other things, he "sette god afore euermore in all his werkis," abstain "fro moche speche," be "nouʒt mich laughyng ne mich playing," and always "vsyng mesure in thingis" (p. 3). Christine de Pizan's list of the qualities of the ideal knight is strikingly similar: he must "aboue all other thyng to loue god," be "of lytyl wordes," "[s]adde in countenaunce," and "amesured and attemporat."[104] Such stringent self-regulation is a requirement for those wishing to enter either the surgical or knightly professions. Impostors who lack these qualities, yet who claim to represent these professions, are frequently attacked by both sorts of writer. Geoffroi de Charny, for example, warns against those who "would prefer to give the appearance of being a good man-at-arms rather than the reality," while Arderne dismisses contemptuously of an impostor who falsely claimed he could heal fistula-in-ano: "at london he deceyued many men" (p. 3).

It is not only through action, but also through discourse, that unfit surgeons can be distinguished from proper ones. This is another respect in which surgical writings converge with their chivalric counterparts. Both knights and surgeons are expected to employ "fair" speech. As the fifteenth-century chivalric prose writer Malory explains, a gentleman may be identified by his use of terms from hunting or other knightly pursuits—by this, "all men of worshyp may discover a jantylman frome a yoman and a yoman frome a vylayne."[105] Similarly, Arderne derides those who use for hemorrhoids terms such as *fics* or *piles*, and insists that "it spedeþ þat lerned men and experte knawe þe maner of spekyng and vse it" (p. 55). His concern with language is technical, but is likely also to do with the social pragmatics of one who clearly expects surgeons to be in aristocratic company, even warning them to be "curtaise at lordeʒ bordeʒ, and displese he noʒt in wordes or dedes to the gestes syttyng by" (p. 6). It is with the aim of impressing such aristocratic elements that he recommends one form of *pulvis sanguis veneris*, an unguent good for the treatment of wounds and ulcers, to the poor, and another, deluxe version to the noble, the latter involving such exotic ingredients as the blood of a young adult virgin. Just as the knight, to return to Lull's words, will often "deffeate a knyght in hym self," so too will many surgeons fail to conform to their own discipline's impossible ideal. As we have seen throughout this study, medieval writers constantly imaged these gaps in identity as wounds in the body. Nowhere is this relationship between body and psyche more pronounced, or more fraught, than in medieval surgery.

Conclusion

In Arderne's treatise on fistula-in-ano, all the qualities that made the medieval body so potent a site of anxiety converge in a single work. The dissolving of the body's form, so contrary to the ideals of order and proportion that governed attitudes both to the body and to society, looms as the central and unfictionalized enemy throughout this anomalous text. At the same time, Arderne's anxious invocation of chivalric tropes throughout his *Practica* gives us insight into the traumatic effects of witnessing such plain reminders of the phantasmatic, and ultimately unstable, nature of identity. Most importantly, however, it shows us that the tensions and traumas of maintaining a chivalric identity inhered not only in its most obvious proponents, such as knights and courtly poets, but within any of those who lived under its stultifying identificatory regime. In the figure of the surgeon, we have a member of medieval society who was often as prominent, as courtly, and as inured to the spectacle of violence as was the knight. For a surgeon like Arderne, whose professional ascendancy hinged upon his toiling in the most transgressive aspects of corporeality, the potential for somatic anxiety increases greatly. This study also, I hope, draws our attention to how this anxiety is not merely a matter of some distant anthropology, but, as is illustrated by the various modern perspectives, as much a part of our own discomfort with the body as it was for medieval writers. Within each of us, competing with our treasured (and imperative) assumptions of stasis and cohesion, is the faint yet nagging fear that we are not, nor ever have been, "hole and sounde."

NOTES

Introduction: Surgery and the Wounds of Sin

1. Quoted in Jack D. Pressman, *Last Resort: Psychosurgery and the Limits of Medicine* (Cambridge and New York: Cambridge University Press, 1998), p. 5.
2. Avicenna, *The Canon of Medicine of Avicenna*, ed. and trans. O. Cameron Gruner (New York: Augustus M. Kelly, 1970), p. 461.
3. Avicenna, *Canon of Medicine of Avicenna*, p. 472.
4. Avicenna, *Canon of Medicine of Avicenna*, p. 474.
5. On the effects of the Fourth Lateran Council, see Carole Rawcliffe, *Medicine and Society in Later Medieval England* (Phoenix Mill: Alan Sutton, 1995; repr. 1997), p. 112 and Nancy Siraisi, *Medieval and Early Renaissance Medicine: An Introduction to Knowledge and Practice*, 1st ed. (Chicago: University of Chicago Press, 1990), pp. 177–78. For the opinion that these effects have been overstated, see Marie-Christine Pouchelle, *The Body and Surgery in the Middle Ages*, trans. Rosemary Morris (New Brunswick, NJ: Rutgers University Press, 1990), pp. 29–30.
6. The proceedings of the Fourth Lateran Council are printed in both Latin and English in *Decrees of the Ecumenical Councils*, ed. Norman P. Tanner, 2 vols. (London: Sheed and Ward, 1990), vol. 1. Canon 18 contains the prohibitions relating to both surgery and torture: "No cleric may decree or pronounce a sentence involving the shedding of blood, or carry out a punishment involving the same, or be present when such punishment is carried out. If anyone, however, under cover of this statute, dares to inflict injury on churches or ecclesiastical persons, let him be restrained by ecclesiastical censure. A cleric may not write or dictate letters which require punishments involving the shedding of blood; in the courts of princes this responsibility should be entrusted to laymen and not to clerics. Moreover no cleric may be put in command of mercenaries or crossbowmen or suchlike men of blood; nor may a subdeacon, deacon or priest practice the art of surgery, which involves cauterising and making incisions; nor may anyone confer a rite of blessing or consecration on a purgation by ordeal of boiling or cold water or of the red-hot iron, saving nevertheless the previously promulgated prohibitions regarding single combats and duels" (p. 244).

7. "All the faithful of either sex, after they have reached the age of discernment, should individually confess all their sins at least once a year, and let them take care to do what they can to perform the penance imposed on them. Let them reverently receive the sacrament of the Eucharist at least at Easter unless they think, for a good reason and on the advice of their own priest, that they should abstain from receiving it for a time. Otherwise they shall be barred from entering a church during their lifetime and they shall be denied a Christian burial at death. Let this salutary decree be frequently published in churches, so that nobody may find the pretence of an excuse in the blindness of ignorance. If any persons wish, for good reasons, to confess their sins to another priest let them first ask and obtain permission of their own priest; for otherwise the other priest will not have the power to absolve or bind them" (*Ecumenical Councils*, 1:245).

8. Mary Flowers Braswell, *The Medieval Sinner* (London: Associated University Presses, 1983), p. 15. Peter Biller, in his excellent introduction to *Handling Sin: Confession in the Middle Ages*, ed. Biller and A.J. Minnis, York Studies in Medieval Theology 2 (York: York Medieval Press, 1998), pp. 3–33, claims that this new frequency of confession led to an unprecedented familiarity between the priest and his flock through the establishment of a "norm, one of individual confessions by parishioners during Lent and their parish priest's careful modulation of penance according to sin and sinner—where the sinner would be well-known to him, and sometimes also the sin" (p. 6).

9. Braswell, *Medieval Sinner*, p. 16.

10. Braswell, *Medieval Sinner*, p. 15.

11. Jerry Root, in his book *"Space to Speke": The Confessional Subject in Medieval Literature* (New York: Peter Lang, 1997), provides an insightful discussion of medieval confession as performance, stressing its status as a lived practice rather than an ordered theological system: "The project of the manuals is to codify and make available a convenient grid, a limited discursive space in which medieval penitents may present themselves. The manuals give a set of prescriptive rules that define and limit this space, but, without exception, they also tie these rules to the promise that confession will permit the penitent to procure access to salvation" (p. 9). The experience of individuality and the pursuit of grace were therefore inextricably linked.

12. Root, *"Space to Speke,"* p. 9.

13. John Myrk, *Myrk's Festial*, ed. Theodor Erbe, Early English Text Society e.s. 96 (1st ed., 1905; repr. Millwood, NY: Kraus Reprint, 1975), p. 2.

14. Joseph Ziegler, *Medicine and Religion c. 1300* (Oxford: Clarendon Press, 1998), p. 9. Ziegler's excellent study also deals with metaphorical intersections between medicine and religion, but his study concentrates on scholastic authorities—and primarily on Arnau de Villanova—and is therefore more concerned with physic than surgery, which was increasingly the domain of artisans rather than of scholars and ecclesiasts.

15. *Ecumenical Councils*, 1:245.

16. *Ecumenical Councils*, 1:245.

17. Guy de Chauliac, *The Cyrurgie of Guy de Chauliac*, ed. M.S. Ogden, Early English Text Society o.s. 265 (London: Oxford University Press, 1971), p. 10.

18. Rawcliffe, *Medicine and Society*, p. 132.

19. See "Scriptorial 'House-Styles' and Discourse Communities," in *Medical and Scientific Writing in Late Medieval English*, ed. Irma Taavitsainen and Päivi Pahta (Cambridge: Cambridge University Press, 2004), pp. 209–40.

20. St. Augustine of Hippo, *The City of God*, trans. Henry Bettenson (New York and London: Penguin Books, 1984), 22:8, pp. 1035–37.

21. R.E. Harvey, *The Inward Wits: Psychological Theory in the Middle Ages and Renaissance* (London: Warburg Institute, 1975), pp. 16–18.

22. Harvey, *Inward Wits*, p. 14.

23. Hildegard of Bingen, *On Natural Philosophy and Medicine*, trans. Margaret Berger (Cambridge: D.S. Brewer, 1999), 3:2, p. 39.

24. Roger Bacon, *The Opus Majus of Roger Bacon*, trans. Robert Belle Burke, 2 vols. (New York: Russell and Russell, 1962), 2:624.

25. Bacon, *Opus Majus*, 2:624.

26. London, British Library MS Sloane 3489, fol. 29r.

27. London, British Library MS Sloane 563, fol. 70r.

28. This dichotomy between "fragmentation and redemption" comes from Caroline Walker Bynum's important book of the same name. I will discuss this idea more fully in chapter 3.

29. John Baldwin, "From the Ordeal to Confession: In Search of Lay Religion in Early Thirteenth-Century France," in *Handling Sin: Confession in the Middle Ages*, ed. Peter Biller and A.J. Minnis, York Studies in Medieval Theology 2 (York: York Medieval Studies, 1998), pp. 198, 205 [191–209].

30. Excerpted in Henry Charles Lea, *The Ordeal*, ed. Edward Peters, with original documents in translation by Arthur E. Howland (Philadelphia: University of Pennsylvania Press, 1973), pp. 186–87.

31. *Jacob's Well*, ed. by Arthur Brandeis, Early English Text Society o.s. 115 (London: K. Paul, Trench, Trübner, 1900), p. 9.

32. *Jacob's Well*, p. 11.

33. *Cursor mundi*, ed. Richard Morris, Early English Text Society o.s. 68, 7 vols. (London: N. Trübner, 1874–93), 5:ll. 23438, 23440.

34. London, British Library MS Sloane 563, fol. 24v.

35. *Fasciculus Morum: A Fourteenth-Century Preacher's Handbook*, ed. and trans. Siegfried Wenzel (University Park and London: Pennsylvania State University Press, 1989), 3:17, pp. 255–57.

36. Faye Getz, in her "Method of Healing in Middle English," in *Proceedings of the 1982 Galen Symposium*, ed. Fridolf Kudlien and Richard J. Durling (Leiden, NY: E.J. Brill, 1991), pp. 147–56, discusses this text in its manuscript context. She dates it at about 1400 and identifies its immediate source as a twelfth-century translation from the Arabic made by Gerard of Cremona (p. 147). Its function in the manuscript, Getz argues, is to supply "the theoretical basis for learned surgery in general, and for wound treatment in particular" (p. 154).

37. London, British Library MS Sloane 6, fols. 202v–303r.

38. John Gaddesden, *Rosa Anglica*, ed. and trans. Winifred Wulff, Irish Text Society 25 (London: Publisher for the Irish Texts Society By Simokin, Marshall, Ltd., 1929 [1923]), p. 53. This text is a translation of an incomplete early modern Irish translation of Gaddesden's Latin text.

39. Berengario da Carpi, *Fracture of the Skull or Cranium*, in Transactions of the American Philosophical Society, vol. 80, pt. 4, ed. L.R. Lind (Philadelphia: American Philosophical Society), p. 68.

40. Berengario da Carpi, *Fracture of the Skull or Cranium*, p. 81.

41. Gaddesden, *Rosa Anglica*, p. 43.

42. London, British Library MS Sloane 3489, fol. 47r.

43. *Speculum Sacerdotale*, ed. Edward H. Weatherly, Early English Text Society o.s. 200 (London: Oxford University Press, 1936), p. 91.

44. Berengario, *Fracture of the Skull or Cranium*, p. 151.

45. London, British Library MS Sloane 3489, fol. 29v.

46. London, British Library MS Sloane 3489, fol. 45r.

47. Lanfranco, *Lanfrank's "Science of Cirurgie,"* ed. Robert v. Fleishhacker, Early English Text Society o.s. 102 (London: Publisher for Early English Text Society by K. Paul, Trench, Trübner, 1894), p. 20.

48. *Of Shrifte and Penance: The Middle English Prose Translation of* Le Manuel Des Péchés, ed. Klaus Bitterling, Middle English Texts 29 (Heidelberg: Carl Winter, 1998), p. 34.

49. London, British Library MS Sloane 6, fol. 199r.

50. London, British Library MS Sloane 6, fol. 199r.

51. London, British Library MS Sloane 277, fol. 22r.

52. Edward Peters, *Torture* (Oxford: Blackwell, 1985), p. 68.

53. Elaine Scarry, *The Body in Pain* (New York: Oxford University Press, 1985), p. 46.

54. John of Arderne, *Treatises of Fistula in Ano*, ed. D'Arcy Power, Early English Text Society o.s. 139 (New York: H. Frowde, 1910), p. 15.

55. *The Book of Vices and Virtues*, ed. W. Nelson Francis, Early English Text Society o.s. 217 (London: Oxford University Press, 1942), p. 176.

56. London, British Library MS Sloane 3489, fol. 37v.

57. *Jacob's Well*, pp. 178–79.

58. John of Arderne, *Treatises*, p. 81.

59. John Trevisa, *On the Properties of Things*, ed. M.C. Seymour, 3 vols. (Oxford: Clarendon Press, 1975–88), 1:438.

60. Lanfranco, *Lanfrank's "Science of Cirurgie,"* p. 107.

61. *Speculum Sacerdotale*, pp. 17–18.

62. *Fasciculus Morum*, 3:17, pp. 255, 257. The comparison of charity to bloodletting was common in confessional manuals. *Jacob's Well*, e.g., argues that excessive wealth is "superfluyte of oþer mennys good'; until we "parte þis good a-sunder" through "blood-letyng," we will remain "syke in synne" (p. 196).

63. Rawcliffe, *Medicine and Society*, pp. 62, 39.

64. London, British Library MS Sloane 240, fol. 7r; New York Academy of Medicine MS 13, fol. 53r.

65. London, British Library MS Sloane 240, fol. 13v.

66. London, British Library MS Sloane 240, fol. 18r.

67. London, British Library MS Sloane 277, fol. 24r.

68. London, British Library MS Sloane 563, fol. 7v.

69. London, British Library MS Sloane 277, fol. 10v.

70. London, British Library MS Sloane 277, fol. 10r.

71. New York Academy of Medicine MS 13, fol. 53r. Guy de Chauliac recommends a similar deception, and attributes its effectiveness to the powers of "contrarie ymaginacioun" (*Cyrurgie*, p. 224). On the manuscripts of Roger Marshall and his misattributed authorship of this anonymous surgery, see Linda Ehrsam Voigts, "Scientific and Medical Books," in *Book Production and Publishing in Britain, 1375–1475*, ed. Jeremy Griffiths and Derek Pearsall (New York: Cambridge University Press, 1989), pp. 345–402.

72. London, British Library MS Additional 30338, fol. 24v.

73. I will discuss Bynum's notion of "fragmentation and redemption" more fully in chapter 3.

Chapter 1   Surgery as Damnation in *Cleanness*

1. These and all subsequent references to *Cleanness* are from *Pearl*-poet, *Sir Gawain and the Green Knight, Pearl, Cleanness, Patience*, ed. J.J. Anderson (London: Dent, 1996).

2. Theresa Tinkle, "The Heart's Eye: Beatific Vision in *Purity*," *Studies in Philology* 85(1998):452[451–70].

3. Tinkle, "Heart's Eye," 457.

4. Sarah Stanbury, *Seeing the "Gawain"-Poet: Description and the Act of Perception* (Philadelphia: University of Pennsylvania Press, 1991), p. 52.

5. Allen J. Frantzen, "The Disclosure of Sodomy in *Cleanness*," *PMLA* 111(1996):452 [451–64].

6. *Decrees of the Ecumenical Councils*, ed. Norman P. Tanner, 2 vols. (London: Sheed and Ward, 1990), 1:243.

7. On this point, see Darrel W. Amundsen, "Medieval Canon Law on Medical and Surgical Practice by the Clergy," *Bulletin of the History of Medicine* 52(1978):22–45.

8. Michael McVaugh, "Therapeutic Strategies: Surgery," in *Western Medical Thought from Antiquity to the Middle Ages*, ed. Mirko D. Grmek et al. (Cambridge, MA: Harvard University Press, 1998), p. 275 [273–290]. McVaugh provides a concise summary of the progress of surgery as a profession from antiquity to the Late Middle Ages.

9. Carole Rawcliffe, *Medicine and Society in Later Medieval England* (Phoenix Mill: Alan Sutton, 1995; repr. 1997), p. 112.

10. Rawcliffe, *Medicine and Society*, p. 112.

11. Quoted in and translated by Magda Pagel-Kroll, "The Surgery of Jamerius: Report on a New Manuscript," *Bulletin of the History of Medicine* 28(1954):477 [471–88].

12. For Augustine's philosophy of the nonsubstance of evil, see his argument against Manichean dualism "Concerning the Nature of the Good," in *Basic Writings of St Augustine*, ed. Whitney J. Oates, trans. P. Holmes (New York: Random House, 1948), pp. 431–57. The actions of humans should be measurable, in keeping with the measure of God, "by whom measure is bestowed on all things"; the failure to act measurably therefore "is justly reprehended for no other cause than that the measure is not there maintained" (p. 439). Evil is simply the absence of moderation and does not itself have any ontological force.

13. St. Augustine of Hippo, "On Nature and Grace," in *Basic Writings of St Augustine*, p. 563.

14. References to such specific medical treatments occur throughout Augustine's writings. Medicine is most frequently used to symbolize the merits of living in accordance with spiritual, rather than worldly, values. Although there is space here only for a few examples, the ubiquity of medical imagery in the work of St. Augustine of Hippo may be illustrated by their high concentration in a single, characteristic text, *Expositions on the Book of Psalms*, trans. J. Tweed and others, 6 vols. (Oxford: J.H. Parker, 1847–57). The technique of binding, which gradually repairs broken or fractured limbs, is often used to illustrate the way in which the convert slowly heals from his or her former, spiritual imbalances: "What are the means whereby He 'bindeth up their bruises?' Just as physicians bind up fractures" (*Expositions*, 6, 147:7, p. 364). Because those who embrace Christ need not fear sickness, they also need not fear its worldly consequences, such as cautery and incision, "the physician's hands with caustics or the knife" (*Expositions*, 1, 6:3, p. 36). Nor is this metaphorics restricted to practical medicine. Augustine will often invoke Galenic theory, such as the following reference to pulse reading: "The Physician had felt his pulse, and knew what was going on within His patient's soul: the patient knew it not" (*Expositions*, 2, 44:19, p. 222). We see, then, that medicine afforded Augustine a wide range of associative possibilities, from the painful (cutting, burning) to the gentle (binding, salves) to the preventative (diagnostic methods).

15. St. Augustine, "On Nature and Grace," p. 523.

16. St. Augustine of Hippo, *Expositions*, 2, 44:14, p. 216.

17. St. Augustine of Hippo, *Expositions*, 1, 34:20, p. 359.

18. "*Temptations*" *from* Ancrene Wisse, ed. Yoko Wada (Osaka: Institute of Oriental and Occidental Studies, Kansai University, 1994), regards homosexuality as the sole "uncundeliche" variety of the "scorpion of lechery," which he or she "ne mei speoken of for scheome" (p. 32). We are told that homosexuality is "so foule and so hidous þat [it] scholde not be nempned" in *The Book of Vices and Virtues* , ed. W. Nelson Francis, Early English Text

Society o.s. 217 (London: Oxford University Press, 1942), p. 46. In each case, sodomy constitutes a linguistic absence; it is not mentioned explicitly, but is designated by its perceived characteristic of being against nature.

19. St. Thomas Aquinas, *Summa Theologiae*, 61 vols. (London: Blackfriars in conjunction with Eyre and Spottiswoode, ca. 1964–81), p. 196. The translation into English is by Martin M. Tweedale, and is quoted in *Basic Issues in Medieval Philosophy*, ed. Richard N. Bosley and Martin M. Tweedale (Peterborough, Ontario: Broadview Press, 1997), p. 573.

20. Isidore of Seville, *Etymologies*, quoted in *A Source Book in Medieval Science*, ed. Edward Grant (Cambridge, MA: Harvard University Press, 1974), p. 701.

21. Lynn Staley Johnson, *The Voice of the* Gawain-*Poet* (Madison, WI: University of Wisconsin Press, 1984), pp. 119, 121.

22. Guy de Chauliac, *The Cyrurgie of Guy de Chauliac*, ed. M.S. Ogden, Early English Text Society o.s. 265 (London: Oxford University Press, 1971), p. 62.

23. *Book of Vices and Virtues*, p. 178.

24. De Chauliac, *Cyrurgie*, p. 62.

25. De Chauliac, *Cyrurgie*, p. 62.

26. John of Arderne, *Treatises of Fistula in Ano*, ed. D'Arcy Power, Early English Text Society o.s. 139 (New York: H. Frowde, 1910), p. 78.

27. *"Temptations" from* Ancrene Wisse, pp. 32, 36.

28. R. Grothé, "Two Middle English Surgical Treatises," unpublished PhD thesis, University of Montreal, 1982, p. 357.

29. De Chauliac, *Cyrurgie*, p. 277.

30. At this point, it could reasonably be objected that neither Lot nor Noah are especially "pure" figures in sacred history. Yet both Noah's nudity before Ham (Genesis 9:23) and Lot's incest (Genesis 19:33, 19:35) are ignored strategically by the poet, in order to contain these characters within a rigidly defined notion of cleanness, in this case a commitment to procreative sexuality. As fecund characters, Noah and Lot are counterpoints to the nonprocreative practices of, respectively, the Predeluvians and the Sodomites. These textual enclosures of the characters within fixed points in their histories relate thematically to the other enclosures in the poem, which connote the purity of those within. As well, we might consider these truncations of biblical history as the poet's own act of "surgery." The poet's selective presentations of Noah and Lot are meant to signify the importance of being "enourled in alle þat is clene" (l. 19). The poet's audience would no doubt have been familiar with these biblical stories in their entireties, and thus they would have understood the point of the poet's manipulation thereof.

31. St. Augustine of Hippo, "On Nature and Grace," p. 535.

32. Frantzen, "Disclosure of Sodomy in *Cleanness*," p. 458.

33. Frantzen, "Disclosure of Sodomy in *Cleanness*," p. 460.

34. For example, see de Chauliac, *Cyrurgie*, p. 276.

35. De Chauliac, *Cyrurgie*, p. 329.

36. De Chauliac, *Cyrurgie*, p. 299.

37. John of Arderne, *Treatises*, p. 20.

38. De Chauliac, *Cyrurgie*, p. 287.

39. De Chauliac, *Cyrurgie*, p. 295.

40. De Chauliac, *Cyrurgie*, p. 300.

41. De Chauliac, *Cyrurgie*, p. 278.

42. *Mandeville's Travels*, ed. M.C. Seymour (London: Oxford University Press, 1968), p. 73.

43. De Chauliac provides a thorough definition of the various types of corrosive medicines and their applications in his *Cyrurgie*, pp. 608–11.

44. For an extended and influential description of cauterization and its various technics, see Albucasis, "On Cauterisation," in *On Surgery and Instruments*, trans. M.S. Spink and G.L. Lewis (Berkeley: University of California Press, 1973), pp. 8-18.

45. Albucasis, *On Surgery and Instruments*, p. 506.

46. John of Arderne, *Treatises*, p. 1.

47. The specific example which Frantzen offers is "the privy into which the little boy is tossed in *The Prioress's Tale*" ("Disclosure of Sodomy in *Cleanness*," p. 460).

48. Juhani Norri, "Notes on the Origin and Meaning of Chemical Terms in Middle English Medical Manuscripts," *Neuphilologische Mitteilungen* 92(1991):223 [215–36].

49. John of Arderne, *Treatises*, p. 86.

50. De Chauliac, *Cyrurgie*, p. 618.

51. Albucasis, *On Surgery and Instruments*, p. 506.

52. Norri, "Notes," p. 222.

53. Lanfranco, *Lanfrank's "Science of Cirurgie,"* ed. Robert v. Fleishhacker, Early English Text Society o.s. 102 (London: Publisher for Early English Text Society by K. Paul, Trench, Trübner, 1894), p. 350.

54. John of Arderne, *Treatises*, p. 81.

55. De Chauliac, *Cyrurgie*, p. 276.

56. John of Arderne, *Treatises*, p. 93.

57. De Chauliac, *Cyrurgie*, p. 611.

58. John of Arderne, *Treatises*, p. 94.

59. John Trevisa, *On the Properties of Things*, ed. M.C. Seymour, 3 vols. (Oxford: Clarendon Press, 1975–88), 1:213.

60. Madeleine Pelner Cosman, "Machaut's Medical Musical World," in *Machaut's World: Science and Art in the Fourteenth Century*, ed. Madeleine Pelner Cosman and Bruce Chandler (New York: New York Academy of Sciences, 1978), p. 6 [1–38].

61. All future references to *Cleanness* will be cited by line number. This passage may also be read as relating to the rulings of the Fourth Lateran Council. According to Lateran IV, as we have seen, priests should not engage in secular callings, nor should a "priest practise the art of surgery, which involves cauterising and making incisions." In *Cleanness*, priests are warned not to "conterfete crafte" (l. 13). "Crafte" can be read as secular activities, such as

surgery, which priests, according to the Fourth Lateran Council, should discard in order to devote their time and energy to spiritual matters. Read this way, the poet implies that, just as Christ cuts bread at Emmaus "blades wythouten" (ll. 1105), so also the priest need not use surgical tools—"as scheres, rasoures and launcetes" (De Chauliac, *Cyrurgie*, p. 4)—to do his job, which is the treatment of spiritual, rather than physical, sickness. Such a reading is in keeping with Francis Ingledew's identification of the poem as "one document among many in late fourteenth-century England to respond aggressively to the condition of the contemporary priesthood, whose perceived uncleanness is the poem's subject," in his "Liturgy, Prophecy, and Belshazaar's Rebellion: Discourse and Meaning in *Cleanness*," *Viator* 23 (1992): 247 [247–79].

62. Pearl-poet, *The Complete Works of the* Pearl-*Poet*, trans. Casey Finch, ed. Malcolm Andrew, Ronald Waldron, and Clifford Peterson (California: University of California Press, 1993), see note for ll. 1105–08 (p. 369).

63. De Chauliac, *Cyrurgie*, p. 9.

64. John of Arderne, *Treatises*, p. 1.

65. Robert J. Blanch and Julian N. Wasserman, *From Pearl to Gawain: Forme to Fynisment* (Gainesville, FL: University Press of Florida, 1995), p. 92. In chapter 4, Blanch and Wasserman discuss the imagery of hands as a metaphor for the relationship between God and humanity, but do not explore the possibility of a medical context.

66. De Chauliac, *Cyrurgie*, p. 2.

67. Lanfranco, *Lanfrank's "Science of Cirurgie*," p. 7.

68. John of Arderne, *Treatises*, p. 6.

69. For example, see T. Millar, "John Arderne, the Father of British Proctology," *Proceedings of the Royal Society of Medicine* 47(1954):6 [75–84].

70. See Nancy Siraisi, *Medieval and Early Renaissance Medicine: An Introduction to Knowledge and Practice* (Chicago: University of Chicago Press, 1990), pp. 177–78.

71. Quoted in Marie-Christine Pouchelle, *The Body and Surgery in the Middle Ages*, trans. by Rosemary Morris (New Brunswick, NJ: Rutgers University Press, 1990), p. 43.

72. See, e.g., Elizabeth B. Keiser, *Courtly Desire and Medieval Homophobia* (New Haven and London: Yale University Press, 1997); Michael Calabrese and Eric Eliason, "The Rhetorics of Pleasure and Sexual Intolerance in *Cleanness*," *Modern Language Quarterly* 56 (1995): 247–75.

73. Grothé, "Two Middle English Surgical Treatises," p. 61.

74. Aristotle, *On the Generation of Animals*, trans. A.L Peck (Cambridge, MA: Harvard University Press, 1963), p. 121.

75. Danielle Jacquart and Claude Thomasset, *Sexuality and Medicine in the Middle Ages*, trans. Matthew Adamson (Princeton, NJ: Princeton University Press, 1988), p. 195.

76. Pseudo-Albertus Magnus, *Women's Secrets*, trans. Helen Rodnite Lemay (Albany: State University of New York Press, 1992), p. 64.

77. Pseudo-Albertus Magnus, *Women's Secrets*, p. 64.

78. Keiser, *Courtly Desire*, p. 3.

79. Calabrese and Eliason, "The Rhetorics," 270.

80. Joan Cadden, *Meanings of Sex Differences in the Middle Ages* (New York: Cambridge University Press, 1993), p. 192.

81. Trevisa, *On the Properties of Things*, 1:306.

82. De Chauliac, *Cyrurgie*, p. 67.

83. Calabrese and Eliason, "The Rhetorics," 254.

84. Calabrese and Eliason, "The Rhetorics," 254.

85. Constantinus Africanus, *De Coitu*, quoted in Paul Delaney, "*De Coitu*: A Translation," *The Chaucer Review* 4:1(1980):56 [55–65].

86. Keiser, *Courtly Desire*, p. 2.

87. Lanfranco, *Lanfrank's "Science of Cirurgie*," p. 174.

88. Calabrese and Eliason, "The Rhetorics," 256; Keiser, *Courtly Desire*, p. 84.

89. Lanfranco, *Lanfrank's "Science of Cirurgie*," p. 173.

Chapter 2   Salvation and *The Siege of Jerusalem*

1. Seymour Fisher and Sidney E. Cleveland, *Body Image and Personality* (New York: Dover Publications, 1968), p. 62.

2. Fisher and Cleveland, *Body Image and Personality*, p. 62.

3. *The Siege of Jerusalem*, ed. E. Kölbing and Mabel Day, Early English Text Society o.s. 188 (Oxford: Oxford University Press, 1932), ll. 840, 1035. All further quotations from the poem will be referenced internally by line number.

4. Caroline Walker Bynum, *Fragmentation and Redemption: Essays on Gender and the Human Body in Medieval Religion* (New York: Zone Books, 1992), pp. 11, 12.

5. Marie-Christine Pouchelle, *The Body and Surgery in the Middle Ages*, trans. Rosemary Morris (New Brunswick, NJ: Rutgers University Press, 1990), pp. 70–87.

6. Pouchelle, *Body and Surgery in the Middle Ages*, p. 75.

7. Bynum, *Fragmentation and Redemption*, p. 272. Bynum states that torturers, unlike surgeons, were not allowed to "sever or divide."

8. Lynn White, Jr., *Medieval Religion and Technology* (Berkeley and London: University of California Press, 1978), p. 331.

9. Carole Rawcliffe, "More Than a Bedside Manner: The Political Status of the Late Medieval Court Physician," in *St George's Chapel in the Late Middle Ages*, ed. Colin Richmond and Eileen Scarff, Historical Monographs Relating to St George's Chapel 17 (Windsor: Dean and Chapter of Windsor, 2001), pp. 77, 79 [71–91].

10. Plato, *Timaeus*, trans. John Warrington (London: Dent, 1965), p. 19 [29d].

11. Plato, *Timaeus*, p. 14 [28].

12. See below for an example of Isidore of Seville's clear use of Ciceronian language to describe the construction of the body.

13. Cicero, *The Nature of the Gods*, trans. P.G. Walsh (Oxford: Clarendon Press, 1997), 2:142, p. 99.

14. Cicero, *Nature of the Gods*, 2:140–41, p. 98; 2:142, p.99.

15. Cicero, *Nature of the Gods*, 2:150, p. 101.

16. Cicero, *Nature of the Gods*, 2:153, p. 103.

17. Cicero, *Nature of the Gods*, 2:153, p. 103.

18. Galen, *On the Usefulness of the Parts of the Body*, trans. Margaret Tallmadge May, 2 vols. (Ithaca, NY: Cornell University Press, 1968), 1:68, 70.

19. St. Ambrose, *Hexameron*, trans. John Savage, Fathers of the Church 42 (Washington: Catholic University Press of America, 1961), 1:5.17, p. 16.

20. St. Augustine of Hippo, *Two Books on Genesis Against the Manichees*, trans. Roland J. Teske (Washington, DC: Catholic University of America Press, 1991), 1:16.26, p. 73.

21. St. Augustine of Hippo, *Two Books*, 1:6.10, pp. 57–58.

22. St. Augustine of Hippo, *Christian Instruction*, trans. John J. Gavignon, Fathers of the Church 4 (Washington: Catholic University of America Press, 1947), 1:19.18, p. 40.

23. St. Augustine of Hippo, *City of God*, 22:24, p. 1072. This chapter of Augustine's great work presents something of a tribute to invention.

24. St. Augustine of Hippo, *Christian Instruction*, 1:30.47, p. 102.

25. John Van Ergen, "Thephilus Presbyter and Rupert of Deutz," *Viator* 2(1980):151 [147–64].

26. Theophilus Presbyter, *De diversis artibus*, trans. C.R. Dodwell (London: Thomas Nelson and Sons, 1961), p. 2.

27. Theophilus Presbyter, *De diversis artibus*, p. 1.

28. Michael Haran, *Medieval Thought*, 2nd ed. (Toronto and Buffalo: University of Toronto Press, 1992), p. 92.

29. Martin Thornton, *English Spirituality* (London: Society for the Propagation of Christian Knowledge, 1963), pp. 110, 108.

30. Thornton, *English Spirituality*, p. 110.

31. Cassiodorus, *Introduction to Divine and Human Letters*, trans. Leslie Webber Jones (New York: Octagon Books, 1966), 1: "Preface," p. 67.

32. Hugh of St. Victor, *The Didascalicon of Hugh of St Victor*, trans. Jerome Taylor (New York: Columbia University Press, 1961), 2:20, p. 74.

33. Hugh of St. Victor, *Didascalicon*, 1:5, pp. 51–52.

34. Hugh of St. Victor, *Didascalicon*, 1:4, p. 51.

35. Hugh of St. Victor, *Didascalicon*, 1:9, pp. 55–56.

36. Hugh of St. Victor, *Didascalicon*, 2:26, p. 78

37. William Caxton, *Caxton's Mirrour of the World*, ed. Oliver H. Prior, Early English Text Society e.s. 110 (London and New York: Oxford Uuniversity Press, 1913 for 1912; repr. 1966), pp. 38–39.

38. Hugh of St. Victor, *Didascalicon*, 1:4, p. 51.

39. Aristotle, *Nichomachean Ethics*, trans. Terence Irwin (Indiana and Cambridge: Hackett, 1985), 1.444:3, p. 10. At 1.441:2, p. 9, Aristotle mocks this theory outright, asking whether being eternal makes a chair more a chair, or a white object whiter.

40. Aristotle, *Nichomachean Ethics*, 1.444:11, p. 12.

41. Aristotle, *Nichomachean Ethics*, 6.32, p. 152.

42. As Roger Bacon argues, speculative science "has the same relation to the other sciences as the science of navigation to the carpenter's art and the military art to the engineer"; it "directs other sciences as its handmaids," just as the mechanical arts are servile to the sciences in their importance to the state. The mechanical arts have no transcendental role in this Aristotelian strain of schematizing knowledge. Roger Bacon, *The Opus Majus of Roger Bacon*, trans. Robert Belle Burke, 2 vols. (New York: Russell and Russell, 1962), 2:633.

43. For an extended discussion of the process by which Platonic rhetoric syn-chaptered with the Aristotelian, see Elspeth Whitney's excellent *Paradise Restored: The Mechanical Arts from Antiquity through to the Thirteenth Century* (Philadelphia: American Philosophical Society, 1990).

44. Bernardus Silvestris, *Commentary on the First Book of Virgil's Aeneid*, trans. Earl G. Schreiber and Thomas E. Maresca (Lincoln and London: University of Nebraska Press, 1979), p. 34.

45. Silvestris, *Commentary*, p. 37.

46. Bonaventure, *De reductione artium ad theologiam*, trans. Sister Emma Thérèse Healy (New York: Saint Bonaventure University, 1955), p. 29.

47. Bonaventure, *De reductione*, p. 21.

48. M.-D. Chenu, *Nature, Man and Society in the Twelfth Century*, ed. and trans. Etienne Gilson (Toronto: University of Toronto Press, 1997), p. 52, footnote 2.

49. Bonaventure, *De reductione*, 1:1, p. 22.

50. Danielle Jacquart, "Medical Scholasticism," in *Western Medical Thought from Antiquity to the Middle Ages*, ed. Mirko D. Grmek (Cambridge, MA: Harvard University Press, 1998), pp. 197–240 (p. 207).

51. Nancy Siraisi, *Medieval and Early Renaissance Medicine: An Introduction to Knowledge and Practice* (Chicago: University of Chicago Press, 1990), p. 180, notes that Guy de Chauliac was able to graduate in both physic and surgery at Bologna, a flexibility not afforded to those studying in northern Europe.

52. However, not all learned practitioners can be shown to have graduated from a university. Some, like Thomas Fayreford, demonstrably attended a medical program without graduating, while others, such as John Arderne, appear never to have attended.

53. Siraisi, *Medieval and Early Renaissance Medicine*, p. 52.

54. Avicenna, *The Canon of Medicine of Avicenna*, ed. and trans. O. Cameron Gruner (New York: Augustus M. Kelly, 1970), p. 20.

55. Lanfranco, *Lanfrank's "Science of Cirurgie,"* ed. Robert v. Fleishhacker, Early English Text Society o.s. 102 (London: Publisher for Early English Text Society by K. Paul, Trench, Trübner, 1894), p. 9.

56. London, British Library MS Sloane 289, fol. 2r.

57. London, British Library MS Sloane 289, fol. 20v.

58. On Galen's attitudes toward surgery, see Michael McVaugh, "Therapeutic Strategies: Surgery," in *Western Medical Thought from Antiquity to the Middle Ages*, ed. Mirko D. Grmek et al. (Cambridge, MA: Harvard University Press, 1998), pp. 275–76.

59. London, British Library MS Sloane 2276, fol. 97r.

60. London, British Library MS Sloane 2276, fols. 102v–103r.

61. Grothè, *Surgical Treatises*, p. 194.

62. John of Mirfield, *Surgery*, ed. James B. Colton (New York: Hafner Publishing Company, 1969), p. 5.

63. London, British Library Harley MS 1736, fol. 8r.

64. On the complex relationship between Bradmore's Latin *Philomena* and Morstede's Middle English derivation, see S.J. Lang, "John Bradmore and his Book *Philomena*," *The Social History of Medicine*, 5 (1992): 121–30. Lang handily refutes R.T. Beck's assertion that Morstede's book is an original vernacular surgery.

65. London, British Library MS Harley 1736, fol. 8r.

66. For another example of the surgeon–carpenter comparison, see Anonymous as edited by Grothè, p. 6.

67. London, British Library MS Harley 1736, fol 9v.

68. Quoted in Pouchelle, *Body and Surgery in the Middle Ages*, p. 43.

69. Pouchelle, *Body and Surgery in the Middle Ages*, p. 43.

70. Elisa Narin Van Court, "*The Siege of Jerusalem* and Augustinian Historians: Writing About Jews in Fourteenth-Century England," *The Chaucer Review* 29:3(1995):229, 231 [227–48].

71. Narin Van Court, "*The Siege of Jerusalem*," p. 232.

72. Narin Van Court, "*The Siege of Jerusalem*," p. 232.

73. Narin Van Court, "*The Siege of Jerusalem*," p. 243.

74. Ralph Hanna III, "Contextualising *The Siege of Jerusalem*," *The Yearbook of Langland Studies* 6 (1992): 112 [109–21].

75. Hanna, "Contextualising *The Siege of Jerusalem*," 115–16.

76. Hanna, "Contextualising *The Siege of Jerusalem*," 114.

77. Narin Van Court, "*The Siege of Jerusalem*," p. 233.

78. White, *Medieval Religion and Technology*, p. 337.

79. Whitney, *Paradise Restored*, p. 111.

80. The library at Llanthony Priory in Gloucestershire, e.g., contained the works of Hugh of St. Victor and Bernardus Silvestris, among others, as well as an entire *armaria* dedicated solely to the writings of St. Augustine. Its Aristotelian holdings were slim in comparison, and built more on the works of natural philosophy than the sciences. See *Libraries of the Austin Canons*, ed. T. Webber and A.G. Watson, Corpus of British Library Catalogues 6 (London: British Library in association with the British Academy, 1998), p. 64 item 229; p. 78 item 350; p. 35; p. 79 item 353.

81. T. Webber and A.G. Watson, "Introduction," in *Libraries of the Austin Canons*, p. 22.

82. See Linda Georgianna, *The Solitary Self: Individuality in the* Ancrene Wisse (Cambridge, MA and London: Harvard University Press, 1981), pp. 12-13.

83. Georgianna, *Solitary Self*, p. 13.

84. Thornton, *English Spirituality*, p. 106.

85. See Reverend J.C. Dickinson, *Origins of the Augustinian Canons and their Introduction into England* (London: Society for the Propagation of Christian Knowledge, 1950), p. 137.

86. Georgianna, *Solitary Self*, p. 14.

87. Georgianna, *Solitary Self*, p. 14.

88. Adam of St. Victor, *The Liturgical Poetry of Adam of St Victor*, trans. Digby S. Wrangham, 3 vols. (Kegan, Paul, Trench: London, 1881), vol. 2, poem 68, pp. 190–91, l. 53; vol. 3, poem 106, pp. 186–87, ll. 8, 12.

89. Dickinson, *Origins of the Augustinian Canons*, p. 138.

90. Chaucer, Geoffrey, *The Canon's Yeoman's Tale*, in *The Riverside Chaucer*, ed. Larry D. Benson, 3rd ed. (Boston: Houghton Mifflin Company, 1987), ll. 992, 993.

91. Jill Mann, *Chaucer and Medieval Estates Satire* (Cambridge: Cambridge University Press, 1973), p. 37.

92. Robert the Scribe, *The Bridlington Dialogue*, trans. a religious of the Community of St. Mary the Virgin (London: Mowbray, 1960), chapter 14, p. 154.

93. Hugh of St. Victor, *Explanation of the Rule of St Augustine*, trans. Dom Aloysius Smith (London: Sands and Company, 1911), p. 80.

94. Carole Rawcliffe, *Medicine for the Soul* (Stroud: Sutton Publishing, 1999), p. 30.

95. Cited in Carole Rawcliffe, *Medicine and Society in Later Medieval England* (Phoenix Mill: Alan Sutton, 1995; repr. 1997), p. 144.

96. Faye Getz, *Medicine in the English Middle Ages* (Princeton, NJ: Princeton University Press, 1998), pp. 50–51.

97. Getz, *Medicine in the English Middle Ages*, p. 51.

98. Carole Rawcliffe, "On the Threshold of Eternity," in *East Anglia's History*, ed. Christopher Harper-Bill, Carole Rawcliffe, and Richard G. Wilson (Bury St Edmunds: Boydell Press, 2002), pp. 46–47 [41–72].

99. See Rudolph Arbesman, "The Concept of 'Christus Medicus' in St Augustine," *Traditio* 10(1954):1–28.

100. St. Augustine of Hippo, "The Rule," in *Augustine of Hippo and his Monastic Rule*, trans. George Lawless (Oxford: Clarendon Press, 1987), 8:1, p. 103.

101. St. Augustine of Hippo, "The Rule," 4:8, p. 91.

102. An example, one of many, is from *Confessions*. Augustine, addressing God, proclaims, "I do not hide my wounds from you. I am sick, and you are the physician." St. Augustine of Hippo, *Confessions*, trans. R.S. Pine-Coffin (London: Penguin Books, 1961), 10:28, p. 232.

103. St. Augustine of Hippo, "The Rule," 5:6, p. 97.

104. St. Augustine of Hippo, "The Rule," 5:6, p. 97.

105. Siraisi, *Medieval and Early Renaissance Medicine*, p. 9.

106. Hugh of St. Victor, *Explanation*, pp. 40, 80.

107. St. Augustine of Hippo, "The Rule," 5:5, p. 97.

108. Phillip Stell, *Medical Practice in Medieval York*, Borthwick Paper 90 (York: University of York, 1996). The following discussion summarises Stell's paper in order to illustrate the ubiquity of surgical treatment in York in the fourteenth century.

109. See Dickinson, *Origins of the Augustinian Canons*, p. 186.

110. *Augustinian Libraries*, p. 90 item 470; p. 420 item 18; p. 333 item 1204.

111. Derek Pearsall, *Old and Middle English Poetry* (London: Routledge, 1977), p. 169.

112. See Stephen K. Wright, *The Vengeance of Our Lord: Medieval Dramatisations of the Destruction of Jerusalem* (Toronto: Pontifical Institute of Medieval Studies, 1989). Regarding the tradition of the Matter of Jerusalem in medieval drama, Wright states, "When we confront the texts in question, our notions of a God of liberation, healing, and reconciliation collide head-on with the image of God as he is presented in the plays: a God who, in the name of divine justice, sanctions enslavement, torture, murder, and merciless revenge" (p. 15).

113. See, e.g., the exemplary collection *An Alphabet of Tales*, ed. Mary M. Banks, Early English Text Society o.s. 126 (London: K. Paul, Trench, Trübner, 1904), pp. 234–35, in which the episode where Josephus heals Titus is proffered as an example of the Christian virtue of forgiveness. See also John Myrk, *Myrk's Festial*, ed. Theodore Erbe, Early English Text Society e.s. 96 (1st ed., 1905; repr. Millwood, NY: Kraus Reprint, 1975), p. 141, where Vespasian, not Titus, meets Nathan and hears his story of Christ's healing miracles; believing this story to be true, Vespasian is cured of the "malady yn hys vysage." Both these works are exhortations to Christian observance, and it is therefore significant that together they invoke the two miraculous healings that occur in *The Siege of Jerusalem*.

114. See Bonnie Millar, *The Siege of Jerusalem in its Physical, Literary, and Historical Contexts* (Dublin: Four Courts Press, 2000), p. 26.

115. *The Northern Passion*, ed. Frances A. Foster (London: K. Paul, Trench, Trübner, 1913 [1912]), ll. 391–92.

116. *Stanzaic Life of Christ*, ed. Frances A. Foster, Early English Text Society o.s. 166 (London: Oxford University Press, 1926), ll. 4278–80.

117. Bonnie Millar, *Siege of Jerusalem*, p. 29.

118. Malcolm Hebron, *The Medieval Siege* (Oxford: Clarendon Press, 1997), p. 134. Hebron's book is a valuable survey and analysis of literary representations of siegecraft in the later Middle Ages, executed in a rigorously historicist mode. Its treatment of *The Siege of Jerusalem*, however, is limited in its view of the poem as strictly a chivalric romance.

119. Hanna, "Contextualising *The Siege of Jerusalem*," p. 112.

120. *Two Old English Apocrypha and their Manuscript Source: The Gospel of Nichodemus and the Avenging of the Saviour*, ed. J.E. Cross (Cambridge: Cambridge University Press, 1997), 1:1, p. 140. The edition I am using contains translations of both the Old English versions of these texts and the Latin originals; all references are to the latter.

121. *Two Old English Apocrypha*, 4:1, p. 160.

122. *Two Old English Apocrypha*, 20:1, p. 208.

123. Eusebius, *Ecclesiastical History*, trans. Lake Kirsopp, 2 vols. (London: William Heinemann, 1926), 1, 85.

124. Eusebius, *Ecclesiastical History*, p. 93.

125. *Two Old English Apocrypha*, p. 250.

126. Jacobus de Voragine, *The Golden Legend* (Hammersmith: Kelmscott Press, 1892), p. 478. All references to Jacobus de Voragine's thirteenth-century *Legenda Aurea* will be to Caxton's Middle English translation.

127. *The Middle English Prose Translation of Roger d'Argenteuil's Bible en François*, ed. Phyllis Moe, Middle English Texts 6 (Heidelberg: Carl Winter, 1977), p. 70. In calling this work "The English Bible," I am following Hebron's practice of referring to the fifteenth-century Middle English translation of Roger d'Argenteuil's *Bible en François* (Hebron, *Medieval Siege*, p. 117). The original French version was a major source for the Jerusalem poems, especially *The Siege of Jerusalem*. Phyllis Moe, in her "The French Source of the Alliterative *Siege of Jerusalem*," *Medium Aevum* 39(1970):147 [147–55], calculates that fully one-third of the poem is taken from the Bible.

128. *Titus and Vespasian*, ed. J.A. Herbert (London: J.B. Nichols, 1905), ll. 1169, 1174.

129. *Sermons from the Worcester Chapter MS, F10*, ed. Dora M. Grisdale, unpublished MA thesis, University of Leeds, 1936, pp. 43, 44.

130. *Of Shrifte and Penance: The Middle English Prose Translation of Le Manuel Des Péchés*, ed. Klaus Bitterling, Middle English Texts 29 (Heidelberg: Carl Winter, 1998), p. 93.

131. Bryon Grigsby, *Pestilence in Medieval and Early Modern Literature* (New York and London: Routledge, 2004), p. 23.

132. Luke Demaitre, "The Description and Diagnosis of Leprosy by Fourteenth-Century Physicians," *Bulletin of the History of Medicine* 59(1985):228 [327–44].

133. Demaitre, "Description and Diagnosis of Leprosy by Fourteenth-Century Physicians," p. 338.

134. Demaitre, "Description and Diagnosis of Leprosy by Fourteenth-Century Physicians," p. 342.

135. Bynum, *Fragmentation and Redempton*, p. 276. Guy de Chauliac lists this resemblance to the dead as one of the signs of leprosy that an examining surgeon should look for before recommending quarantine. Shared characteristics between leprous and dead bodies include "foule coloure, morphe, scabbe and stinkynge filþes" (*The Cyrurgie of Guy de Chauliac*, ed. M.S. Ogden, Early English Text Society o.s. 265 [London: Oxford University Press, 1971], p. 379).

136. John Trevisa, *On the Properties of Things*, ed. M.C. Seymour, 3 vols. (Oxford: Clarendon Press, 1975–88), 1:426. De Chauliac, too, attributes some cases of leprosy not to "contagiouse," but to "heritage" (*Cyrurgie*, p. 383).

137. *Two Old English Apocrypha*, p. 244.

138. De Chauliac, *Cyrurgie*, p. 3.

139. Eve Kuryluk, *Veronica and her Cloth: History, Symbolism and Structure of a "True" Image* (Oxford: Oxford University Press, 1991), p. 7.

140. Translated by John Shinners in *Medieval Popular Religion, 1000–1500: A Reader*, ed. John Shinners (Peterborough: Broadview Press, 1997), p. 286,

originally in Latin in Tony Hunt, *Popular Medicine in Thirteenth-Century England* (Cambridge: D.S. Brewer, 1990), pp. 27–28.

141. Rawcliffe, *Medicine and Society*, p. 94.

142. George R. Keiser, *A Manual of the Writings in Middle English*, 10, ed. Albert E. Hartung, (New Haven: Connecticut Academy of Arts and Sciences), p. 3672.

143. York, York Minster MS 16.E.32, fol. 129r.

144. *Speculum Christiani*, ed. Gustaf Holmstedt, Early English Text Society o.s. 182 (London: Oxford University Press, 1933 [1929]), p. 182.

145. Narin van Court, "*The Siege of Jerusalem*," p. 231.

146. Narin van Court, "*The Siege of Jerusalem*," p. 231.

147. *Middle English Sermons*, ed. Woodburn O. Ross, Early English Text Society o.s. 209 (Oxford: Oxford University Press, 1940 for 1938), p. 126.

148. Stell, *Medical Practice*, p. 7.

149. From the materials compiled by John Flint South, *Memorials of the Craft of Surgery in England*, ed. D'Arcy Power (London: Cassell and Company, Limited, 1886), p. 297.

150. Although the subsequent tradition of Christian historiography would assimilate Josephus into its own religious context, Josephus never himself converted, and he frequently defended Judaism in his writings. This, despite the fact that he was viewed by the Jews as a traitor, and was, for the remainder of his life, in favor with Vespasian and the Romans. See Samuel S. Kottek, *Medicine and Hygiene in the Works of Flavius Josephus* (Leiden and New York: E.J. Brill, 1994), pp. 3–5.

151. Josephus, *The Jewish Wars*, ed. and trans. S. Gaalya Cornfeld et al. (Tel Aviv: Massade, 1982), p. 232.

152. John Trevisa, *The English Polychronicon*, ed. Richard A. Seeger, 2 vols., unpublished PhD chapter, University of Washington, 1975, 1:420. Trevisa completed his translation in the 1380s, which could well have been consulted by the *Siege*-poet.

153. Kottek, *Medicine and Hygiene*, p. 24.

154. Bonnie Millar, *Siege of Jerusalem*, p. 65.

155. De Chauliac, *Cyrurgie*, p. 10.

156. London, British Library MS Sloane 277, fols. 22v, 11r.

157. On the debate over wound treatment in medieval surgery, see Pouchelle, *Body and Surgery in the Middle Ages*, pp. 58–59. Pouchelle astutely notes that the disagreement as regards the appropriate level of surgical interference when healing a wound is not merely a medical matter, but suggests a broader cultural and theological concern with the purity of the body: "Refusing to allow the wound to suppurate meant forcing the sufferer to 'reabsorb' and 'digest' the malign forces which had him in their grip. This internalisation could not be accepted without a change in mental attitudes which was scarcely likely to be effected by the sight of a purely technical improvement in efficiency."

158. De Chauliac, in his *Cyrurgie*, p. 10, dismisses those surgeons, such as Theodoric of Cervia, who "drieden indifferently alle woundes wiþ wyne

alone," and those like William de Saliceto who "procureden alle woundes wiþ swete oynementis and emplastres."

159. Extract trans. M. Teresa Tavormina, "Henry of Lancaster, *The Book of Holy Medicine*," in *Cultures of Piety*, ed. Anne Clark Bartlett and Thomas H. Bestul (Ithaca: Cornell University Press, 1999), p. 26 [19–40].

160. *Medical Writings of the Fourteenth Century*, ed. George Henslow (London: Chapman and Hall, 1899), pp. 48–49.

161. See Getz, *Medicine in the English Middle Ages*, p. 41.

162. Rawcliffe, *Medicine and Society*, p. 95.

163. *Riverside Chaucer*, p. 30, ll. 413–30.

164. Chaucer lists "Bernard, and Gatesden, and Gilbertyn" (l. 434), all of whom included charms in their treatises.

165. *Riverside Chaucer*, p. 72, ll. 3480, 3483.

166. *Riverside Chaucer*, p. 307, l. 603; p. 308, l. 606.

167. Rawcliffe, *Medicine and Society*, p. 126.

168. See Getz, *Medicine in the English Middle Ages*, p. 44.

169. Getz, *Medicine in the English Middle Ages*, p. 41.

170. *Libraries of the Augustinian Canons*, p. 325 item 1168; p. 420 item 16; p. 325 item 1169.

171. Peter Murray Jones, "Thomas Fayreford: An English Fifteenth-Century Medical Practitioner," in *Medicine from the Black Death to the French Disease*, ed. Roger French et al. (Ashgate: Aldershot, 1998), p. 177 [156–83].

172. Cited in Pouchelle, *Body and Surgery in the Middle Ages*, p. 53.

173. Moses Maimonedes, *Moses Maimonedes' Two Treatises on the Regimen of Health*, ed. and trans. Ariel Bar-Sela et al. (Philadelphia: American Philosophical Society, 1962), p. 25.

174. *The Siege of Jerusalem* is not as explicit in its terminology regarding the use of contraries as the other versions of the story. *The Golden Legend*, although it does not designate Josephus a medical practitioner, nonetheless has him "rememberyng that contraryes ben cured by theyr contraryes" (p. 480).

175. See above, n108.

176. For a discussion of this motif in early penitential literature, see *Medieval Handbooks of Penance*, ed. John T. McNeill and Helena M. Gamer (New York: Columbia University Press, 1990), pp. 44–45.

177. St. Augustine of Hippo, *Christian Instruction*, 1:14.13, pp. 36–37.

178. London, British Library Sloane MS 277, fol. 49r.

179. In his introduction to his edition of the poem, p. 9, Foster notes that the poet uses both the *Polychronicon* and the *Legenda Aurea* as sources. We have already seen how the *Polychronicon* is used in *The Siege of Jerusalem*. *The Golden Legend* was also a source for the *Siege*-poet, and most clearly for the episode where Titus is cured of his paralysis.

180. William Caxton, *The Game of Chess*, facsimile from the copy of Trinity College, Cambridge (London: Scholar Press, 1976), p. 110.

181. Lanfranco, *Lanfrank's "Science of Cirurgie,"* p. 33.

182. Lanfranco, *Lanfrank's "Science of Cirurgie,"* p. 34.
183. Lanfranco, *Lanfrank's "Science of Cirurgie,"* p. 34.
184. Lanfranco, *Lanfrank's "Science of Cirurgie,"* p. 32.
185. Lanfranco, *Lanfrank's "Science of Cirurgie,"* p. 32.
186. For a discussion of this arming scene, see A.C. Spearing, *Readings in Medieval Poetry* (Cambridge: Cambridge University Press, 1987), p. 168. Spearing argues that the poet "renders the scene fully into art, with an intertwining of gray steel and bright gold, metals symbolic respectively of warfare and of royal luxury," demonstrating an appreciation of the poet's flair for visual framing.
187. Trevisa, *On the Properties of Things*, 1:285.
188. Trevisa, *On the Properties of Things*, 1:287.
189. Jacobus de Voragine, *Golden Legend*, p. 40.
190. Trevisa, *On the Properties of Things*, 1:243, 268, 272.
191. Isidore of Seville, "Isidore of Seville: The Medical Writings," trans. William D. Sharpe, in *Transactions of the American Philosophical Society* 54(1964):40–41.
192. Trevisa, *On the Properties of Things*, 1:230.
193. Vitruvius, *The Ten Books on Architecture*, trans. Morris Hicky Morgan, 2nd ed. (New York: Dover Publications, 1960), 1:2.4, p. 14.
194. See Paul Frankl, *The Gothic*, on medieval architectural theory and aesthetics (pp. 86–110).
195. Lanfranco, *Lanfrank's "Science of Cirurgie,"* p. 19.
196. Vitruvius, *Ten Books on Architecture*, Book 6, p. 167.
197. Vitruvius, *Ten Books on Architecture*, 1:1.10, p. 10.
198. Frankl, *Gothic*, p. 103.
199. Teresa Grace Frisch, *Gothic Art, 1140–c.1450: Sources and Documents* (Englewood Cliffs: Prentice-Hall, 1971), p. 25.
200. Frisch, *Gothic Art*, p. 26.
201. Frisch, *Gothic Art*, p. 34.
202. *English Fragments from Latin Medieval Service-Books*, ed. Henry Littlehales, Early English Text Society e.s. 90 (London: K. Paul, Trench, Trübner, 1903), pp. 6–7.
203. Dickinson, *Origins of the Augustinian Canons*, p. 71.
204. Fisher and Cleveland, *Body Image and Personality*, p. 351.

Chapter 3   The Priest: John Audelay's Wounds of Sin

1. For the most important work to date on the Audelay manuscript, Oxford, Bodleian Library MS Douce 302, see Susanna Fein, "Good Ends in the Audelay Manuscript," *Yearbook of English Studies* 33 (2003): 97-119. Fein argues convincingly that Audelay oversaw the production of the manuscript from first to last, working with a redactor and a compiler, and divides its content into four sections: the unified work *The Counsel of Conscience*, Salutations and Prayers, Carols, and a "meditative close" (99).

158 NOTES

2. The date and title of this work and the vocation of its author we know from
the colophon that appears at the end of the *Concilium*: "*Finito libro: sit launs
et gloria. Christo liber vocatur: concilium consciencie, sic nominatur scala celi: et vita
salutis eterni. Iste liber compositus per Johannem Awdelay capellanum qui fuit secus
et surdus in sua visitacione. Ad honorem domini nostri Jhesu Christi. Et ad exem-
plum aliorum in monasterio de Haghmon. Anno domini millesimo cccc visecimo vj.
Cuius anime propicietur deus Amen*" (p. 149). This and all subsequent references to John Audelay's book are taken from the standard edition of
Audelay's poems, *The Poems of John Audelay*, ed. Ella Keats Whiting, Early
English Text Society o.s. 184 (London: Oxford University Press, 1931), and
will be cited internally by line number.
3. William Langland, "Prologue," in *The Vision of Piers the Plowman*, ed.
A.V.C. Schmidt (New York: Everyman, 1995), l. 98; Audelay, *Poems of
John Audelay*, 2.240.
4. See Nicholas Watson, "Censorship and Cultural Change in Late-Medieval
England," *Speculum* 70(1995):823 [822–63]. According to Watson, "the
term 'vernacular theology' is intended as a catchall, which in principle could
include any kind of writing, sermon, or play that communicates theological
information to the audience." Audelay's sweeping overview of various
pastoral and devotional commonplaces fits perfectly into this description.
5. Watson, "Censorship and Cultural Change in Late-Medieval England,"
p. 827.
6. Richard Firth Green, "Marcolf the Fool and Blind John Audelay," in
Speaking Images: Essays in Honor of V.A. Kolve, ed. Charlotte Morse and
Robert F. Yeager (Asheville, NC: Pegasus Press, 2001), p. 567 [559–76];
James Simpson, *Reform and Cultural Revolution: The Oxford English Literary
History Volume 2: 1350–1547* (Oxford and New York: Oxford University
Press, 2002), p. 380. For the satiric strategies of this poem see
James Simpson, "Saving Satire after Arundel's *Constitutions*: John
Audelay's 'Marcol and Solomon,' " in *Text and Controversy from Wyclif to
Bale*, ed. Helen Barr and Ann Hutchison (Turnhout: Brepols, 2005),
pp. 387–404.
7. Keating, "Introduction," p. xiv.
8. Green, "Marcolf the Fool," p. 565.
9. Tim William Machan, *Textual Criticism and Middle English Texts*
(Charlottesville and London: University Press of Virginia, 1994), p. 104.
10. Eric G. Stanley, "The True Counsel of Conscience, or The Ladder of
Heaven: In Defense of John Audelay's Unlyrical Lyrics," in *Expedition der
Wahrheit*, ed. Stefan Horlacher and Marion Islinger (Heidelberg: Carl
Winder Universitätsverlag, 1996), p. 137 [131–59].
11. Arthur Kleinman, *The Illness Narratives* (USA: Basic Books, 1987), p. 48.
12. Michael Bennett, "John Audelay: Some New Evidence of his Life and
Work," *The Chaucer Review* 16:4(1982):353 [344–55].
13. Bennett, "John Audelay," 347.
14. Critics seem divided on the merit of Bennett's thesis as an explanation for
Audelay's highly admonitory voice. Green finds Audelay's autobiographical

moments rather too general to refer to "so dramatic an act" (Green, "Marcolf the Fool," p. 566), while Susanna Fein accepts that the incident of 1417 "seems to have had a scarring effect" (Fein, "Good Ends," p. 100).

15. The proceedings of the Fourth Lateran Council are printed in both Latin and English in *Decrees of the Ecumenical Councils*, ed. Norman P. Tanner, 2 vols. (London: Sheed and Ward, 1990). The passage reads, "All the faithful of either sex, after they have reached the age of discernment, should individually confess all their sins at least once a year, and let them take care to do what they can to perform the penance imposed on them. Let them reverently receive the sacrament of the Eucharist at least at Easter unless they think, for a good reason and on the advice of their own priest, that they should abstain from receiving it for a time. Otherwise they shall be barred from entering a church during their lifetime and they shall be denied a Christian burial at death. Let this salutary decree be frequently published in churches, so that nobody may find the pretence of an excuse in the blindness of ignorance. If any persons wish, for good reasons, to confess their sins to another priest let them first ask and obtain permission of their own priest; for otherwise the other priest will not have the power to absolve or bind them" (I:245).

16. *Middle English Religious Prose*, ed. N.F. Blake (London: E. Arnold, 1972), p. 72. Moira Fitzgibbons has argued that this work, an ecclesiastically sanctioned translation of an authoritative Latin catechism, signals a turning point in "vernacular theology" by managing to "advocate a new form of spiritual authority for laypeople" through its avoidance of the rhetorical complexity of much surrounding Middle English sermonic writing. See her "Disruptive Simplicity: Gaytryge's Translation of Archibishop Thoresby's *Injunctions*," in *The Vernacular Spirit*, ed. Renate Blumenfeld-Kosinski et al. (New York: Palgrave, 2002), p. 41 [39–57].

17. Marjorie Curry Woods and Rita Copeland, "Classroom and Confession," in *The Cambridge History of Medieval English Literature*, ed. David Wallace (Cambridge and New York: Cambridge University Press, 1999), pp. 389–91 [376–406].

18. *Middle English Religious Prose*, p. 75.

19. See Robert R. Raymo, "Works of Religious and Philosophical Instruction," in *A Manual of Writings in Middle English 1050–1500*, ed. Albert E. Hartung (New Haven: Connecticut Academy of Arts and Sciences, 1986), p. 2267.

20. *Book to a Mother*, ed. Adrian James McCarthy, Elizabethan and Renaissance Studies 92 (Salzburg: Institut für Anglistik und Amerikanistik, Universität Salzburg, 1981), p. 71.

21. William Caxton, *Quattuor Sermones*, ed. N.F. Blake (Heidelberg: Carl Winter, 1974), p. 24.

22. Nicholas Orme, *Medieval Children* (New Haven:Yale University Press, 2001), pp. 81–82.

23. *Clensyng of Mannes Sowle*, ed. Walter Kennedy Everett, unpublished PhD thesis, University of North Carolina at Chapel Hill, 1974, p. 3; Caxton, *Quattuor Sermones*, p. 63.

24. John Myrk, *Myrk's Festial*, ed. Theodor Erbe (1st ed., 1905; repr. Millwood, NY: Kraus Reprint, 1975), p. 171.

25. *The Mirroure of the Worlde*, ed. Robert R. Raymo and Elaine Whitaker, Medieval Academy Books 106 (Toronto: University of Toronto Press, 1990), p. 54.

26. Nicholas Love, *Nicholas Love's Mirror of the Blessed Life of Jesus Christ*, ed. Michael Sargent (New York: Garland Publishing, 1992), p. 10. For the argument that Love's program of meditations is a conservative treatise designed to actively repress lay theology, see Watson, "Censorship and Cultural Change in Late-Medieval England," p. 853. For the opposing point of view-that Love's book empowers readers to imagine scriptural episodes beyond the limits circumscribed by the Church-see Simpson, *Reform and Cultural Revolution*, p. 442.

27. *Book to a Mother*, p. 62.

28. Watson, "Censorship and Cultural Change in Late-Medieval England," p. 836.

29. Watson, "Censorship and Cultural Change in Late-Medieval England," p. 835.

30. Tanner, *Ecumenical Councils*, canon 22, 1:245.

31. *The Middle English "Mirror,"* ed. Kathleen Marie Blumreich (Arizona: Arizona Center for Medieval and Renaissance Studies, 2002), p. 365.

32. London, British Library MS Sloane 3489, fol. 30v.

33. London, British Library MS Sloane 3489, fol. 29r.

34. *Go, Crysten Soul: A Critical Edition of* The Crafte of Dying, ed. Mary Etta Scott, unpublished PhD thesis, Miami University, 1975, p. 157.

35. R. Grothé, "Two Middle English Surgical Treatises," unpublished PhD thesis, University of Montreal, 1982, p. 357.

36. *Middle English "Mirror,"* p. 441, 294.

37. *þe Pater Noster of Richard Ermyte: A Late Middle English Exposition of the Lord's Prayer*, ed. Flor Aarts, editor's proefschrift (Nijmegen: Drukkerij Gebr., Janssen, 1967), p. 14. This witty observation on the misplaced priorities of parishioners demonstrates what Raymo has aptly referred to as this writer's "broad human sympathies" and pragmatic concerns with rhetorical "simplicity and lucidity" (Raymo, "Works of Religious and Philosophical Instruction," p. 2281).

38. *The Household of Edward IV*, ed. A.R. Meyers (Manchester: Manchester University Press, 1959), pp. 124–25.

39. Printed in *Medieval Handbooks of Penance*, ed. John T. McNeill and Helena M. Gamer (New York: Columbia University Press, 1990), p. 251.

40. Translated in Woods and Copeland, "Classroom and Confession," p. 386.

41. William Caxton, *Ryall Booke* (London: Rycharde Pynson, 1507), chapter 99.

42. Theodoric of Cervia, *The Surgery of Theodoric*, trans. Eldridge Campbell and James Colton, 2 vols. (New York: Appleton-Century-Crofts, 1960), 1:4.

43. On the problem of overenthusiastic penitents, especially according to Jean Gerson, see Dyan Elliot, "Women and Confession," in *Gendering the Master Narrative*, ed. Mary C. Erler and Maryanne Kowaleski (Ithaca and London: Cornell University Press, 2003), p. 45 [31–51].

44. *Speculum Vitae*, ed. John W. Smeltz, unpublished PhD thesis, Duquesne University, 1977, l. 8189.

45. *Fasciculus Morum: A Fourteenth-Century Preacher's Handbook*, ed. and trans. Siegfried Wenzel (University Park and London: Pennsylvania State University Press, 1989), 3:17, p. 256.

46. Green, "Marcolf the Fool," pp. 567, 566.

47. Simpson, *Reform and Cultural Revolution*, p. 380.

48. Whiting, "Íntroduction," p. xiv.

49. Fein, "Good Ends," p. 104.

50. Fein, "Good Ends," p. 107.

51. *The Book of Tribulation*, ed. Alexandra Barratt (Heidelberg: Carl Winter, 1983), p. 52.

52. *Book of Tribulation*, p. 59.

53. *Go, Crysten Soul*, pp. 208, 205.

54. Printed in *Yorkshire Writers*, ed. C. Horstman, 2 vols. (London: Swan Sonnenschein, 1896), 2:450. According to Raymo in his *Manual*, the *De Visitacione infirmorum* tradition was not only rhetorical but practical, "widely used by priests in ministering to the dying as part of the rite known as The Visitation of the Sick, which included prayer, exhortation, and interrogation, as well as the sacraments of Penance, the Eucharist, and Extreme Unction" (p. 2360). Audelay, himself a chantry priest as well as a sufferer, may have both given and received this rite before dictating this poem.

55. Kleinman, *Illness Narratives*, p. 32.

56. Kleinman, *Illness Narratives*, p. 27.

57. Fein, "Good Ends," p. 2, fn 2.

58. Benvenutus Grassus, *The Wonderful Art of the Eye*, ed. L.M. Eldredge (East Lansing: Michigan State University Press, 1996), p. 58.

59. Stanley, "The True Counsel of Conscience," p. 143.

60. Simpson, *Reform and Cultural Revolution*, p. 440.

61. The *salutacio Sancte Brigitte*, which celebrates the founding of Syon Abbey in 1415, is poem 23 in Whiting's edition.

62. Gail McMurray Gibson, *The Theater of Devotion* (Chicago and London: The University of Chicago Press, 1989), p. 7.

63. Gibson, *Theater of Devotion*, p. 6.

64. Fein, "Good Ends," p. 115.

65. *Pore Caitif*, ed. Sister Mary Teresa Brady, unpublished PhD thesis, Fordham University, 1954, p. 12.

66. *Quatrefoil of Love*, ed. Israel Gollancz and Magdalene M. Weale, Early English Text Society o.s. 195 (London: Oxford University Press, 1935), ll. 499–500.

67. *The Prickynge of Love*, ed. Harold Kane, Elizabethan and Renaissance Studies 92:10, 2 vols. (Salzburg: Institute für Anglistik und Amerikanistik: Universität Salzburg, 1983), 1:168.

68. Richard Rolle, *Richard Rolle: Prose and Verse*, ed. S.J. Ogilvie-Thomson, Early English Text Society o.s. 293 (Oxford: Oxford University Press, 1988), p. 75.

69. "An Autumn Song," in *Religious Lyrics of the Fourteenth Century*, ed. Carleton Brown, Reverend G.V. Summers, 2nd ed. (Oxford: Clarendon Press, 1924), ll. 29–35.

70. *Clensynge of Mannes Soule*, ed. Walter Kennedy Everett, unpublished PhD thesis, University of North Carolina at Chapel Hill, 1974, pp. 84–85.

71. *Speculum Vitae*, ll. 37–38.

72. *Middle English "Mirror,"* pp. 1–2.

73. Roger Dalrymple, *Language and Piety in Middle English Romance* (Cambridge and Rochester: D.S. Brewer, 2000), p. 18.

74. John Lydgate, *The Siege of Thebes*, Early English Text Society o.s. 108, 125, 2 vols. (London: Oxford University Press, 1960), 1:ll. 2388–2404.

75. London, British Library MS Sloane 277, fol. 22v.

76. Grothé, "Two Middle English Surgical Treatises," p. 430.

77. Muriel Joy Hughes, *Woman Healers in Medieval Life and Literature* (Freeport: Books for Libraries Press, 1968).

78. *Eger and Grime*, ed. James Ralston Caldwell (Cambridge: Harvard University Press, 1933), ll. 216, 218. Subsequent references will appear as line numbers in the text.

79. For the work of this official painter to the city of Brussels, see Dirk De Vos, *Roger Van Der Weyden: The Complete Works* (New York: Harry N. Abrams, 1999).

80. See, e.g., the depiction of the Harrowing of Hell from *Quatrefoil of Love*, where David celebrates the liberation of the Old Testament patriarchs by playing his harp:

> For his haly handwerke heried he helle,
> And all broghte he oute of bale þat euer hade bene his;
> Dauyd, his derlynge, made myrthe þer emelle,
> He tuk an harpe in his hande and weldide it iwysse;
>
> (ll. 261–64)

81. *A Devout Tretryse Called The Tree, & xii Frutes of the Holy Ghost*, ed. J.J. Vaissier (Groningen: Wolters, 1960), p. 29; *Prickynge of Love*, 1:192.

82. Other examples of female pietas depicting a woman bemoaning the spectacle of the wounded male hero in the presence of the surgeon can be found in the romance tradition. See, e.g., *Sir Tryamour*:

> That lady sorowed in hur wede
> When sche sawe hur sone blede,
> That all wan was hur blee and hur blode.
> Tryamowre kyssed hys modur in hye
> And seyde, "Modur, let be yowre crye;
> Me eylyth nothyng but gode."
> A leche was sent aftur in that stownde
> For to serche the chyldys wounde
> And for to stawnche the chyldys blode.
> Tryamowre he undurtoke belyve
> To save hym upon hys lyfe,
> Then mendyd hys modurs mode.
>
> (ll. 904–15)

This scene greatly resembles descriptions of Mary sorrowing before Christ on the cross, and incorporates the surgeon, or "leche," who heals the hero's wound in a context far removed from the penitential "wounds of sin" imagery that dominated didactic religious writings. *Sir Tryamour* has been edited in *Four Middle English Romance*, ed. Harriet Hudson (Kalamazoo: Medieval Institute Publications, 1996).

83. Henry Laughlin, *The Ego and its Defenses* (New York: Appleton-Century-Crofts, 1970), p. 172.

84. *A Myrour to Lewde Men and Wymmen*, ed. Venetia Nelson (Heidelberg: Carl Winter, 1981), pp. 163–64.

85. *Myrour to Lewde Men and Wymmen*, p. 164.

86. *The Doctrinal of Sapience*, ed. Joseph Gallagher, Middle English Texts 26 (Heidelberg: Universitätsverlag Carl Winter), p. 107.

87. Whiting, "Introduction," p. xviii.

88. Quoted in James W. Jones, *Contemporary Psychoanalysis and Religion* (New Haven:Yale University Press, 1991), p. 9.

89. Sigmund Freud, "The Dynamics of Transference," in Sigmund Freud, *The Standard Edition of the Complete Psychological Works of Sigmund Freud*, ed. And trans. James Strachey et al. (London: Hogarth Press, 1953–74), 12:104. For a passionate and eloquent defense of the use of psychoanalysis to explicate medieval texts and culture, see Louise O. Fradenburg, "Be Not Far From Me: Psychoanalysis, Medieval Studies and the Subject of Religion," *Exemplaria* 7:1(1995):41–54. In this article, Fradenburg argues against the positivist insistence from within medieval studies that the only way to understand the literature of the Middle Ages is to identify with its writers on their terms has prevented us from benefiting from the same methodologies that illuminate human societies in our own time. This insistence, she argues, is founded on the refusal to acknowledge "the ways in which medieval culture might have misunderstood itself," and also the attribution to the Middle Ages of a false integrity that ignores "the construction of subjectivity as an historical process" (p. 45).

90. Leo B. Thomas, "Sacramental Confession and Some Clinical Concerns," *Journal of Religion and Health* 4:4(1965):351 [345–53]. Conversely, some Catholic writers have vehemently opposed the rise of psychoanalysis as a competing form of therapy to auricular confession. For example, Andreas Snoeck, in his *Confession and Psychoanalysis*, trans. Theodore Zuydwijk, Maryland: Newman Press, 1964, urges the creation of a "Christian analysis," one that takes into account that "suffering is a profound mystery, the solution of which does not lie within [the psychoanalyst's] province but in God's redemptive love" (p. 82).

91. Myrk, *Myrk's Festial*, p. 2.

92. Quoted in James W. Jones, *Contemporary Psychoanalysis*, p. 31.

93. William Caxton, *The Doctrinal of Sapience*, ed. Joseph Gallagher, Middle English Texts 26 (Heidelberg: Universitätsverlag Carl Winter), p. 116.

94. Sigmund Freud, *Introductory Lectures on Psychoanalysis* (England: Penguin, 1991).

95. Julia Kristeva, *Powers of Horror: An Essay on Abjection*, trans. Léon S. Roudiez (New York: Columbia University Press, 1982), p. 71.

96. *Anchoritic Spirituality: Ancrene Wisse and Associated Works*, trans. Anne Savage and Nicholas Watson, Classics of Western Spirituality 73 (New York: Paulist Press, 1991), p. 129.

97. "The Middle English St. Brendan's Confession," ed. R.H. Bowers, *Archiv* 175(1939):44 [40–49]. According to Raymo in the *Manual*, the attribution to St. Brendan is spurious (p. 2359). For an illuminating discussion of stench and excrement as conventional attributes of the iconography of Hell, see Thomas L. Seiler, "Filth and Stench as Aspects of the Iconography of Hell," in *The Iconography of Hell*, ed. Clifford Davidson and Thomas L. Seiler (Kalamazoo: Medieval Institute Publications, 1992), pp. 132–40. Seiler demonstrates that the biblical imagery of "oderiferous brimstone" (p. 132) in Genesis inaugurates a tradition by which malodor signifies both sin and its punishments and which found experiential reinforcement in the very real experience of stench and filth of the busy urban centers of the later Middle Ages.

98. Melanie Klein, *Our Adult World and Other Essays* (New York: Basic Books, 1963), p. 26.

99. "Stans puer ad mensam," in *The Babees Book*, ed. Frederick J. Furnivall, Early English Text Society o.s. 72 (London: K. Paul, Trench, Trübner, 1868), pp. 262–63.

100. "John Drury and his English Writings," ed. Sanford Brown Meech, *Speculum* 9(1934):82 [70–83].

101. Dan Michel, *Dan Michel's Ayenbite of Inwit*, Early English Text Society o.s. 23 (London: K. Paul, Trench, Trübner, 1866), pp. 52, 84, 135.

102. *Myrour to Lewde Men and Wymmen*, p. 79.

103. *The Book of Vices and Virtues*, ed. W. Nelson Francis, Early English Text Society o.s. 217 (London: Oxford University Press, 1968), p. 98.

104. *Yorkshire Writers*, 2:436; *Mirroure of the Worlde*, p. 123.

105. Caxton, *Quattuor Sermones*, p. 53.

106. *Myrour to Lewde Men and Wymmen*, p. 146.

107. Kristeva, *Powers of Horror*, 72.

108. Cited in James W. Jones, *Contemporary Psychoanalysis and Religion*, p. 58.

109. *The Chastising of God's Children*, ed. Joyce Bazire and Eric Colledge (Oxford: Blackwell, 1957), p. 113.

110. *Chastising of God's Children*, pp. 113, 115.

111. John L. Fleming, "Nonpharmacological Methods for Dealing with Preoperative Anxiety," in *Emotional and Psychological Responses to Surgery*, ed. Frank Guerra and J. Antonio Aldrete (Grune and Strattoni: New York, 1980), p. 42 [37–45].

112. *Chastising of God's Children*, p. 145.

113. *Yorkshire Writers*, p. 451.

114. John Trevisa, *On the Properties of Things*, ed. by M.C. Seymour, 3 vols. (Oxford: Clarendon Press, 1975–88), 1:438.

115. William of Shoreham, "The Seven Sacraments," in *The Poems of William of Shoreham*, ed. M. Konrath, Early English Text Society e.s. 86 (1902; repr. Oxford: Oxford University Press, 1975), pp. 1–78, ll. 967–74.
116. Kleinman, *Illness Narratives*, p. 26.

Chapter 4   The Surgeon: Surgery, Chivalry, and Sin in the *Practica* of John Arderne

1. John of Arderne, *Treatises of Fistula in Ano*, ed. D'Arcy Power, Early English Text Society o.s. 139 (New York: H. Frowde, 1910), p. 1; citations in the text to the *Practica* refer to the page number of this edition.
   The Middle English version edited by Power is perfect for my argument, since it limits itself to the details of Arderne's surgical practice, discarding the more general medical material of the Latin *Practica*. Peter Murray Jones notes in his essay "Four Middle English Translations of John Arderne," in *Latin and Vernacular*, ed. A.J. Minnis (Cambridge: D.S. Brewer, 1989), pp. 61–89 that this Middle English version was designed as "a systematic exposition of Arderne on fistula-in-ano and related subjects" (p. 72); in Jones's view, this material suffers little degradation of meaning from the Latin original, since the translator "succeeds remarkably" in capturing its sense (p. 81). I will also cite, where they are available, Middle English versions of other treatises on medicine and chivalry, whether French, Italian, or Latin. Thus this chapter will explore the views of the body available in the secular world of England in this period.
2. On the exaltedness of Arderne's clientele, see Peter Murray Jones, "Four Middle English Translations of John Arderne," p. 65. For the definitive critique of the most commonly made insubstantiated claims about Arderne's life-that he was educated at Montpellier, worked for John of Gaunt, went on military campaigns, and died in 1390-see Huling E. Ussery, *Chaucer's Physician: Medicine and Literature in Fourteenth-Century England*, Tulane Studies in English 19 (New Orleans: Faculty of English of Tulane University, 1971), pp. 62–69.
3. Kathleen Kelly, "Malory's Body Chivalric," *Arthuriana* 6:4(1996):54 [52–71].
4. *MED*, 1168, s.v. dissolve.
5. Jeffrey Jerome Cohen, *Of Giants*, Medieval Cultures 17 (Minneapolis: University of Minnesota Press, 1999), p. 81.
6. Jacques Lacan, "The Mirror Stage," in *Écrits: A Selection*, trans. Alan Sheridan (New York: W.W. Norton, 1977), pp. 1–7 (p. 4).
7. Jacques Lacan, "Aggressivity in Psychoanalysis," in *Écrits: A Selection*, p. 11 [8–29].
8. Cohen, *Of Giants*, p. 68.
9. Cohen (and the members of Inscripta), "The Armour of an Alienating Identity," *Arthuriana* 6:4(1996):2 [1–24].

10. Kelly, "Malory's Body Chivalric," 54.

11. Kelly, "Malory's Body Chivalric," 64.

12. T. Millar, "John Arderne, the Father of British Proctology," *Proceedings of the Royal Society of Medicine* 47(1954):75 [75–84].

13. St. Augustine of Hippo, "Concerning Order," excerpted in *Basic Issues in Medieval Philosophy*, ed. Richard N. Bosley and Martin Tweedale (Peterborough, Ontario: Broadview Press, 1997), pp. 518–19.

14. St. Augustine of Hippo, "Concerning Order," p. 519.

15. Cicero, *The Nature of the Gods*, trans. P.G. Walsh (Oxford: Clarendon Press, 1997), 2:141, p. 98.

16. Carole Rawcliffe, *Sources for the History of Medicine in Late Medieval England* (Kalamazoo: Medieval Institute Publications, 1995), p. 31.

17. It is precisely because of fistula-in-ano's extreme effects that this condition is used, throughout the history of writing, to depict the vulnerability of the flesh. In the Old Testament, e.g., God chooses this condition as the most effective means by which to punish the disobedient Israelites, giving them "the ulcer of Egypt" that afflicts the place "by which the dung is cast out, with the scab and the itch" (Deuteronomy 28:7). St. Augustine of Hippo, in *The City of God*, trans. Henry Bettenson (New York and London: Penguin Books, 1984), 22:8, tells of the counselor Innocentius, who, when "under treatment for fistulas, having a number of them intertwined in the rectum, and others more deep-seated," was cured not by worldly medicine, but by the prayers of holy men. Of Chaucer, it has been argued by David Williams in "Radical Therapy in the Miller's Tale," *The Chauer Review* 15(1981):227–35 that Absalon's branding of Nicholas with the hot poker is a parody of the operation for cauterizing fistula-in-ano, and is meant to lend force to the branding as a punishment for Nicholas's excessive venality. In the early modern period, we find in book 3 of Spenser's *The Faerie Queene* (London: Dent, 1987) the lovelorn heroine Britomart comparing her fleshly pangs to "bleeding bowells" in which "th'ulcer groweth daily more and more" (3:2.39). Also in the early modern period, in Shakespeare's comedy *All's Well That Ends Well*, we find a French king suffering from a fistula whose location is never specified, but which Bard C. Cosman argues is fistula-in-ano; see Bard C. Cosman, "All's Well That End's Well: Shakespeare's Treatment of Anal Fistula," *Diseases of the Colon and Rectum* 41:7(1998):914–24. This brief survey of the image of anal fistula in pre-Enlightenment literature should leave us with the impression that, in looking for a condition that best represents the pathology of the body, fistula-in-ano was often first in the literary imagination.

18. Didier Anzieu, *Skin Ego* (London: Karnac, 1989), p. 38.

19. Anzieu, *Skin Ego*, p. 39.

20. William S. Haubrich, *Medical Meanings: A Glossary of Word Origins* (Philadelphia, PA: American College of Physicians, 1997), p. 90.

21. Elizabeth Grosz, *Volatile Bodies* (Bloomington: Indiana University Press, 1994), p. 39.

22. Grosz, *Volatile Bodies*, p. 79.

23. Grosz, *Volatile Bodies*, p. 80.

24. Grosz, *Volatile Bodies*, p. 100.

25. Georges Bataille, *L'érotisme* (1962); see Georges Bataille, *Eroticism*, trans. Mary Dalwood (London: Boyars, 1987), p. 17.

26. "Isidore of Seville: The Medical Writings," trans. William D. Sharpe, *Transactions of the American Philosophical Society* 54 (1964): 45.

27. Quoted in Marie-Christine Pouchelle, *The Body and Surgery in the Middle Ages*, trans. Rosemary Morris (New Brunswick, NJ: Rutgers University Press, 1990), p. 147.

28. Quoted in Linda Paterson, "Military Surgery: Knights, Serjeants and Raimon of Avignon's Version of the *Chirurgia* of Roger of Salerno (1180–1209)," in *Ideals and Practice of Medieval Knighthood 2*, ed. Christopher Harper-Bill et al. (Suffolk: Boydell Press, 1986), pp. 117–46 (p. 124).

29. R. Grothé, "Two Middle English Surgical Treatises," unpublished PhD thesis, University of Montreal, 1982, p. 125.

30. Guillaume de Deguileville, *The Pilgrimage of the Lyfe of the Manhode*, ed. Avril Henry, Early English Text Society o.s. 288, 2 vols. (London: Oxford University Press, 1985), 1:ll. 5701–02, 5536.

31. Grothé, "Two Middle English Surgical Treatises," p. 118.

32. Mary Douglas, *Purity and Danger: An Analysis of Concepts of Pollution and Taboo* (London: Routledge and Kegan Paul, 1966), p. 35.

33. Douglas, *Purity and Danger*, p. 38.

34. Roy Porter, *The Greatest Benefit to Mankind* (London: Fontana Press, 1999), p. 84.

35. Grothé, "Two Middle English Surgical Treatises," p. 357.

36. Douglas, *Purity and Danger*, p. 121.

37. Luke Demaitre, "Medieval Notions of Cancer: Malignancy and Metaphor," *Bulletin of the History of Medicine* 72(1998):620 [609–37].

38. *Bestiary*, trans. Richard Barber (Woodbridge: Boydell Press, 1992), p. 148.

39. Theodoric of Cervia, *The Surgery of Theodoric*, trans. Eldridge Campbell and James Colton, 2 vols. (New York: Appleton-Century-Crofts, 1960), 1:115.

40. Peter Murray Jones, "John Arderne and Surgery," in *Practical Medicine from Salerno to the Black Death*, ed. Luis García-Ballester et al. (Cambridge: Cambridge University Press, 1994), p. 307 [289–321].

41. Albucasis, *On Surgery and Instruments*, trans. M.S. Spink and G.L. Lewis (Berkeley: University of California Press, 1973), pp. 502–11.

42. Theodoric's section on anal fistulas is in his *Surgery of Theodoric*, pp. 115–18.

43. Medical historians have retrospectively considered Arderne's instruments cumbersome, and even inimical to the precision such an operation requires; see Nancy Siraisi, *Medieval and Early Renaissance Medicine: An Introduction to Knowledge and Practice* (Chicago: University of Chicago Press, 1990), p. 185.

44. Carole Rawcliffe, *Medicine and Society in Later Medieval England* (Phoenix Mill: Alan Sutton, 1995; repr. 1997), p. 112. As previously noted, Darrel W. Amundsen in "Medieval Canon Law on Medical and Surgical Practice by the Clergy," *Bulletin of the History of Medicine* 52(1978) cautions

against exaggerating the influence of such edicts, stressing that they were limited to the very highest orders of clergy.

45. Pouchelle, *Body and Surgery in the Middle Ages*, p. 24.

46. Julia Kristeva, *Powers of Horror: An Essay on Abjection*, trans. Léon S. Roudiez (New York: Columbia University Press, 1982), p. 71.

47. Lanfranco, *Lanfrank's "Science of Cirurgie,"* p. 208.

48. John Trevisa, *On the Properties of Things*, ed. M.C. Seymour, 3 vols. (Oxford: Clarendon Press, 1975–88), 2:1302.

49. Avicenna, *The Canon of Medicine of Avicenna*, ed. and trans. O. Cameron Gruner (New York: Augustus M. Kelly, 1970), p. 42.

50. Thomas Norton, *Ordinal of Alchemy*, ed. John Reidy, Early English Text Society o.s. 272 (London: Oxford University Press, 1975), ll. 2007, 2014.

51. Trevisa, *On the Properties of Things*, 2:1339.

52. Richard Palmer, "In Bad Odour: Smell and its Significance in Medicine from Antiquity to the Seventeenth Century," in *Medicine and the Five Senses*, ed. W.F. Bynum and Roy Porter (Cambridge: Cambridge University Press, 1993), p. 66 [61–68].

53. Kristeva, *Powers of Horror*, p. 72.

54. Bataille, *Eroticism*, p. 17.

55. Bataille, *Eroticism*, p. 58.

56. Bataille, *Eroticism*, p. 57.

57. Bataille, *Eroticism*, p. 82.

58. Guy de Chauliac, *The Cyrurgie of Guy de Chauliac*, ed. M.S. Ogden, Early English Text Society o.s. 265 (London: Oxford University Press, 1971), p. 4.

59. Grothé, "Two Middle English Surgical Treatises," p. 545.

60. *Pearl-poet, Sir Gawain and the Green Knight, Pearl, Cleanness, Patience*, ed. J.J. Anderson (London: Dent, 1996), cited internally by line number.

61. On Isidore's etymology and medieval definitions of surgery, see Michael McVaugh, "Therapeutic Strategies: Surgery," in *Western Medical Thought from Antiquity to the Middle Ages*, ed. Mirko D. Grmek et al. (Cambridge, MA: Harvard University Press, 1998), pp. 273–90.

62. Christine de Pizan, *The Book of Fayttes of Armes and of Chyvalrye*, trans. William Caxton, ed. A.T.P. Byles, Early English Text Society o.s. 189 (London: Oxford University Press, 1937), p. 21.

63. De Pizan, *Book of Fayttes of Armes*, pp. 38–39.

64. *Of Arthour and of Merlin*, ed. O.D. Macrae-Gibson, Early English Text Society o.s. 268, 2 vols. (London: Oxford University Press, 1979), 2:ll. 6043–44.

65. Quoted in Paterson, "Military Surgery," p. 138.

66. Grothé, "Two Middle English Surgical Treatises," p. 478.

67. Ramon Lull, *The Book of the Ordre of Chyualry*, trans. William Caxton, ed. A.T.P. Byles, Early English Text Society o.s. 168 (London: Oxford University Press, 1999), p. 102.

68. Lull, *Book of the Ordre of Chyualry*, p. 35.

69. Avicenna, *Avicenna's Tract on Cardiac Drugs and Essays on Arab Cardiotherapy*, ed. Hakeem Abdul Hameed (Pakistan: Handard Foundation Press, 1983), p. 38.

70. Avicenna, *Avicenna's Tract on Cardiac Drugs*, p. 22.

71. Lull, *Book of the Ordre of Chyualry*, p. 15.

72. Geoffroi de Charny, *The Book of Chivalry of Geoffroi de Charny*, ed. and trans. Richard Kaeuper and Elspeth Kennedy (Philadelphia: University of Pennsylvania Press, 1996), p. 177.

73. Lull, *Book of the Ordre of Chyualry*, p. 70.

74. *Knyghthode and Bataile*, ed. R. Dyboski and Z.M. Arend, Early English Text Society o.s. 201 (London: Oxford University Press, 1935), ll. 369–75. Cited in the text by line number.

75. For example, the fifteenth-century lyric "Jesus woundes so wide" (from British Library Arundel MS Arundel 286), connects the Son's "woundes so wide" to "welles of lif to the goode." See R.T. Davies, *Medieval English Lyrics* (London: Faber and Faber, 1963), p. 216, ll. 1–2.

76. Rawcliffe, *Medicine and Society*, p. 137. Such measures were taken not only for the corporeal remnants of surgical procedures but also for those of other trades involving organic material, such as butchery. E.L. Sabine, in "Butchering in Mediaeval London," *Speculum* 8 (1933): 335–53, documents the measures taken by officials in medieval London to curb unhygienic disposal practices by the city's butchers. According to Sabine, bad meats were described as, e.g., "putrid and stinking, an abomination to mankind" (p. 339). It was made illegal to carelessly discard bad meats—as well as hair, teeth, and gristle—in legislation created not only by city officials, but also by the king himself in writs issued in 1369, 1370, and 1371 (p. 345). This anxiety with which "corrupt" organic matter was described and treated in this period may be compared to the regulations to which barbers were subject. Both professions invoked sensations of horror due to their shared status as reminders of (what Lacan would call) the Real, the unbounded manner in which the body is first experienced.

77. The documents cited in this paragraph are printed in *Memorials of the Craft of Surgery in England*, from materials compiled by John Flint South, ed. D'Arcy Power (London: Cassell and Co., 1886), p. 297.

78. *Memorials of the Craft of Surgery*, pp. 301–302.

79. *Memorials of the Craft of Surgery*, p. 318.

80. Lull, *Book of the Ordre of Chyualry*, pp. 63–64.

81. Judith Butler, *Bodies That Matter* (New York: Routledge, 1993), p. 9.

82. De Chauliac, *Cyrurgie*, p. 13.

83. *The Squire of Low Degree*, in *Middle English Verse Romances*, ed. Donald Sands (Exeter: University of Exeter Press, 1986), pp. 249–78, ll. 255, 183.

84. Lull, *Book of the Ordre of Chyualry*, p. 78.

85. *Lanterne of Liȝt*, ed. Lilian M. Swinburn, Early English Text Society o.s. 151 (London: K. Paul, Trench, Trübner, 1917), p. 65. While the *Lanterne of Liȝt* is, strictly speaking, more of a religious treatise than a chivalric one, it does

contain much lamenting of the current state of knighthood and concerns itself with offering more appropriate models of behavior. In this way, it is a valuable resource for attitudes toward knighthood in the period. It is worth noting, as well, that this image of the girdle from *Lanterne of Li3t* retains its appeal as a metaphor for the durability of Christian virtue far beyond the fifteenth century. Matthew Arnold's 1867 poem "Dover Beach," e.g., also images faith as an enclosing girdle, only to illustrate the extent to which this metaphorical garment had loosened in his own time:

The Sea of Faith
Was once, too, at the full, and round earth's sphere
Lay like the folds of a bright girdle furl'd.
But now I only hear
Its melancholy roar,
Retreating, to the breath
Of the night-wind, down the vast edges drear
And naked shingles of the world.

(ll. 21–28)

See *The Poetical Works of Matthew Arnold*, ed. C.B. Tinker and H.E. Lowry (London: Oxford University Press, 1950).

86. London, Wellcome Institute Library, MS Wellcome 799, fol. 16r.
87. London, Wellcome Institute Library, MS Wellcome 799, fol. 16r.
88. Cohen, *Of Giants*, pp. 67–68.
89. Cohen, *Of Giants*, p. 68.
90. Theodoric of Cervia, *Surgery of Theodoric*, pp. 196–97; my italics here and throughout this paragraph.
91. Grothé, "Two Middle English Surgical Treatises," p. 412.
92. Cohen, *Of Giants*, p. 105.
93. M.M. Bakhtin, *The Dialogic Imagination*, ed. Michael Holquist, trans. Caryl Emerson and Michael Holquist (Austin: University of Texas Press, 1981), pp. 153–54.
94. Grosz, *Volatile Bodies*, p. 38.
95. De Charny, *Book of Chivalry*, p. 101.
96. De Charny, *Book of Chivalry*, p. 103.
97. De Charny, *Book of Chivalry*, p. 193.
98. For an extended discussion of the interdependence of bodies and garments in Old French courtly literature in relation to the theories of Elizabeth Grosz, see E. Jane Burns, "Speculum of the Courtly Lady," *Journal of Medieval and Early Modern Studies* 29:2(Spring 1999):253–92.
99. Butler, *Bodies That Matter*, p. 3.
100. De Charny, *Book of Chivalry*, pp. 122–23.
101. Lull, *Book of the Ordre of Chyualry*, p. 33.
102. *The Household of Edward IV*, ed. A.R. Meyers (Manchester: Manchester University Press, 1959), p. 124.

103. Court was not the only place in which a surgeon could identify with the knightly persona. As Ruth Mazo Karras has shown in "Sharing Wine, Women, and Song: Masculine Identity Formation in the Medieval European Universities," in *Becoming Male in the Middle Ages*, ed. Jeffrey Jerome Cohen and Bonnie Wheeler (New York: Garland Publishing, 1997), pp. 187–202, student bodies at European universities (which would include the famous Continental medical schools) were primarily comprised of a "social elite," the members of which often carried weapons and dressed in a fashion that "echoe[d] ideals of heroic masculinity" (pp. 189–90).

104. De Pizan, *Book of Fayttes of Armes*, p. 23.

105. Thomas Malory, "Isolde the Fair," in *The Works of Sir Thomas Malory*, ed. Eugène Vinaver, 2nd ed. (Oxford: Clarendon Press, 1971), pp. 229–74 (p. 232).

BIBLIOGRAPHY

Manuscripts

British Library, Additional MS 30338; Harley MS 1736; Sloane MSS 6, 240, 277, 289, 563, 3489.
New York Academy of Medicine MS, 13.
Wellcome Institute Library, Wellcome MS, 799.
York Minster MS, 16.E.32.

Primary Sources

A Devout Tretryse Called The Tree, & xii Frutes of the Holy Ghost, ed. J.J. Vaissier (Groningen: Wolters, 1960).
A Myrour to Lewde Men and Wymmen, ed. Venetia Nelson (Carl Winter: Heidelberg, 1981).
A Source Book in Medieval Science, ed. Edward Grant (Cambridge, MA: Harvard University Press, 1974).
Adam of St. Victor, *The Liturgical Poetry of Adam of St Victor*, trans. Digby S. Wrangham, 3 vols. (London: K. Paul, Trench, Trübner, 1881).
Alain de Lille, *The Plaint of Nature*, trans. James J. Sheridan (Toronto: Pontifical Institute of Medieval Studies, 1980).
Albucasis, *On Surgery and Instruments*, trans. M.S. Spink and G.L. Lewis (Berkeley: University of California Press, 1973).
An Alphabet of Tales, Early English Text Society o.s. 126–27, ed. Mary M. Banks (London: K. Paul, Trench, Trübner, 1904).
Anchoritic Spirituality: Ancrene Wisse and Associated Works, trans. Anne Savage and Nicholas Watson, Classics of Western Spirituality 73 (New York: Paulist Press, 1991).
Aristotle, *Nicomachean Ethics*, trans. Terence Irwin (Indiana and Cambridge: Hackett, 1985).
———, *On the Generation of Animals*, trans. A.L. Peck (Cambridge: Harvard University Press, 1963).
Audelay, John, *The Poems of John Audelay*, ed. Ella Keats Whiting, Early English Text Society o.s. 184 (London: Oxford University Press, 1931).
Avicenna, *The General Principles of Avicenna's Canon of Medicine*, trans. Mazhar H. Shah (Karachi: Naveed Clinic, 1966).

Avicenna, *Avicenna's Tract on Cardiac Drugs and Essays on Arab Cardiotherapy*, ed. Hakeem Abdul Hameed (Pakistan: Handard Foundation Press, 1983).

Bacon, Roger, *The Opus Majus of Roger Bacon*, trans. Robert Belle Burke, 2 vols. (New York: Russell and Russell, 1962).

Basic Issues in Medieval Philosophy, ed. Richard N. Bosley and Martin M. Tweedale (Peterborough, Ontario: Broadview Press, 1997).

Bestiary, trans. Richard Barber (Woodbridge: Boydell Press, 1992).

Bonaventure, *De reductione artium ad theologiam*, trans. Sister Emma Thérèse Healy (New York: Saint Bonaventure University, 1955).

The Book of Tribulation, ed. Alexandra Barratt (Heidelberg: Carl Winter, 1983).

The Book of Vices and Virtues, ed. W. Nelson Francis, Early English Text Society o.s. 217 (London: Oxford University Press, 1942).

Book to a Mother, ed. Adrian James McCarthy, Elizabethan and Renaissance Studies 92 (Salzburg: Institut für Anglistik und Amerikanistik, Universität Salzburg, 1981).

Cassiodorus, *Introduction to Divine and Human Letters*, trans. Leslie Webber Jones (New York: Octagon Books, 1966).

Caxton, William, *Caxton's Mirrour of the World*, ed. Oliver H. Prior, Early English Text Society, e.s. 110 (1913 for 1912; repr. London and New York: Oxford University Press, 1966).

———, *The Doctrinal of Sapience*, ed. Joseph Gallagher, Middle English Texts 26 (Heidelberg: Universitätsverlag C. Winter).

———, *The Game of Chess*, facsimile from the copy at Trinity College, Cambridge (London: Scholar Press, 1976).

———, *Quattuor Sermones*, ed. N.F. Blake (Heidelberg: Winter, 1974).

———, *Ryall Booke* (London: Rycharde Pynson, 1507).

The Chastising of God's Children, ed. Joyce Bazire and Eric Colledge (Oxford: Blackwell, 1957).

Cicero, *The Nature of the Gods*, trans. P.G. Walsh (Oxford: Clarendon Press, 1997).

Clensyng of Mannes Sowle, ed. Walter Kennedy Everett, unpublished PhD thesis (University of North Carolina at Chapel Hill, 1974).

Cultures of Piety, ed. Anne Clark Bartlett and Thomas H. Bestul (Ithaca: Cornell University Press, 1999).

Cursor Mundi, ed. Richard Morris, Early English Text Society o.s. 68, 7 vols. (London: K. Paul, Trench, Trübner, 1874–93).

De Charny, Geoffroi, *The Book of Chivalry of Geoffroi de Charny*, ed. and trans. Richard Kaeuper and Elspeth Kennedy (Philadelphia: University of Pennsylvania Press, 1996).

De Chauliac, Guy, *The Cyrurgie of Guy de Chauliac*, ed. M.S. Ogden, Early English Text Society o.s. 265 (London: Oxford University Press, 1971).

Decrees of the Ecumenical Councils, ed. Norman P. Tanner, 2 vols. (London and Washington: Sheed and Ward and Georgetown University Press, 1990).

De Deguileville, Guillaume, *The Pilgrimage of the Lyf of the Manhode*, ed. Avril Henry, Early English Text Society o.s. 288, 2 vols. (London: Oxford University Press, 1985).

Delany, Paul, Constantinus Africanus's *De Coitu*: A Translation, *The Chaucer Review*, 4(1970):55–65.

De Pizan, Christine, *The Book of Fayttes of Armes and of Chyvalrye*, trans. William Caxton, ed. A.T.P. Byles, Early English Text Society o.s. 189 (London: Oxford University Press, 1937).

Eger and Grime, ed. James Ralston Caldwell (Cambridge: Harvard University Press, 1933).

English Fragments from Latin Medieval Service-Books, ed. Henry Littlehales, *Early English Text Society* e.s. 90 (London: K. Paul, Trench, Trübner, 1903).

Eusebius, *Ecclesiastical History*, trans. Lake Kirsopp, 2 vols. (London: William Heinemann, 1926).

Fasciculus Morum: A Fourteenth-Century Preacher's Handbook, ed. and trans. Siegfried Wenzel (University Park and London: Pennsylvania State University Press, 1989).

Four Middle English Romance, ed. Harriet Hudson (Kalamazoo: Medieval Institute Publications, 1996).

Frisch, Teresa Grace, *Gothic Art, 1140-c.1450: Sources and Documents* (Englewood Cliffs: Prentice-Hall, 1971).

Gaddesden, John, *Rosa Anglica*, ed. and trans. Winifred Wulff, Irish Text Society 25 (1929 for 1923).

Galen, *On the Usefulness of the Parts of the Body*, trans. Margaret Tallmadge May, 2 vols. (New York: Cornell University Press, 1968).

Go, Crysten Soul: A Critical Edition of The Crafte of Dying, ed. Mary Etta Scott, unpublished PhD thesis (Miami University, 1975).

Grassus, Benvenutus, *The Wonderful Art of the Eye: A Critical Edition of the Middle English Translation of his "De probatissima arte oculorum,"* ed. L.M. Eldredge (East Lansing: Michigan State University Press, 1996).

Grothé, R., *Two Middle English Surgical Treatises*, unpublished PhD thesis (University of Montreal, 1982).

Hildegard of Bingen, *On Natural Philosophy and Medicine*, trans. Margaret Berger (Cambridge: D.S. Brewer, 1999).

The Household of Edward IV, ed. A.R. Meyers (Manchester: Manchester University Press, 1959).

Hugh of St. Victor, *The Didascalicon of Hugh of St Victor*, trans. Jerome Taylor (New York: Columbia University Press, 1961).

———, *Explanation of the Rule of St Augustine*, trans. Dom Aloysius Smith (London: Sands and Company, 1911).

Isidore of Seville, "Isidore of Seville: The Medical Writings," trans. William D. Sharpe, in *Transactions of the American Philosophical Society*, 54(1964):5–75.

Jacob's Well, ed. Arthur Brandeis, Early English Text Society o.s 115 (London: K. Paul, Trench, Trübner, 1900).

Jacobus de Voragine, *The Golden Legend* (Hammersmith: Kelmscott Press, 1892).

"John Drury and His English Writings," ed. Sanford Brown Meech, *Speculum*, 9(1934):70–83.

John of Arderne, *Treatise of Fistula in Ano*, ed. D'Arcy Power, Early English Text Society o.s. 139 (New York: H. Frowde, 1910).

John of Mirfield, *Surgery*, ed. James B. Colton (New York: Hafner Publishing Company, 1969).

John Scotus Eriugena, *Periphyseon*, trans. I.P. Sheldon-Williams, rev. John J. O'Meara (Washington: Dumbarton Oaks, 1987).

Josephus, *The Jewish Wars*, ed. and trans. S. Gaalya Cornfeld et al. (Tel Aviv: Massade, 1982).

Knyghthode and Bataile, ed. R. Dyboski and Z.M. Arend, Early English Text Society o.s. 201 (London: Oxford University Press, 1935).

Lanfrank, *Science of Cirurgie*, ed. Robert V. Fleischhacker, Early English Text Society o.s. 102 (New York: C. Scribner and Co., 1894).

Langland, William, *The Vision of Piers the Plowman*, ed. A.V.C. Schmidt (New York: Everyman, 1995).

Lanterne of Liÿt, ed. Lilian M. Swinburn, Early English Text Society o.s. 151 (London: K. Paul, Trench, Trübner, 1917).

Lawless, George, *Augustine of Hippo and his Monastic Rule* (Oxford: Clarendon Press, 1987).

Love, Nicholas, *Nicholas Love's Mirror of the Blessed Life of Jesus Christ*, ed. Michael Sargent (New York: Garland Publishing, 1992).

Lull, Ramon, *The Book of the Ordre of Chyualry*, trans. William Caxton, ed. A.T.P. Byles, Early English Text Society o.s. 168 (London: Oxford University Press).

Lydgate, John, *The Siege of Thebes*, Early English Text Society o.s. 108, 125, 2 vols. (London: Oxford University Press, 1960).

Maimonedes, Moses, *Moses Maimonedes' Two Treatises on the Regimen of Health*, ed. and trans. Ariel Bar-Sela et al. (Philadelphia: American Philosophical Society, 1964).

Malory, Thomas, *The Works of Sir Thomas Malory*, ed. Eugène Vinaver, 2nd ed. (Oxford: Clarendon Press, 1971).

Mandeville's Travels, ed. M.C. Seymour (London: Oxford University Press, 1968).

Maurus of Salerno, *Optimus Physicus*, in *Transactions of the American Philosophical Society*, ed. Morris Harold Saffron, 62:1(1972).

Medical Writings of the Fourteenth Century, ed. George Henslow (London: Chapman and Hall, 1899).

Medieval Handbooks of Penance, ed. John T. McNeill and Helena M. Gamer (New York: Columbia University Press, 1938; repr. 1990).

Medieval Popular Religion, 1000–1500: A Reader, ed. John Shinners (Peterborough, Ontario: Broadview Press, 1997).

Memorials of the Craft of Surgery in England, from materials compiled by John Flint South, ed. D'Arcy Power (London: Cassell and Co., 1886).

Michel, Dan, *Dan Michel's Ayenbite of Inwit*, Early English Text Society o.s. 23 (London: K. Paul, Trench, Trübner, 1866).

The Middle English "Mirror," ed. Kathleen Marie Blumreich (Arizona: Arizona Center for Medieval and Renaissance Studies, 2002).

The Middle English Prose Translation of Roger d'Argenteuil's Bible en François, ed. Phyllis Moe, Middle English Texts 6 (Heidelberg: Winter, 1977).

Middle English Religious Prose, ed. N.F. Blake (London: E. Arnold, 1972).

Middle English Sermons, ed. Woodburn O. Ross, Early English Text Society o.s. 209 (Oxford: Oxford University Press, 1940).

"The Middle English St. Brendan's Confession," ed. R.H. Bowers, *Archiv*, 175(1939):40–49.

The Mirroure of the Worlde, ed. Robert R. Raymo and Elaine Whitaker, Medieval Academy Books 106 (Toronto: University of Toronto Press, 1990).

Myrk, John, *Myrk's Festial*, ed. Theodor Erbe, Early English Text Society e.s. 96 (1905; repr. Millwood, NY: Kraus Reprint, 1975).

Norton, Thomas, *The Ordinal of Alchemy*, ed. John Fischer, Early English Text Society o.s. 272 (London: Oxford University Press, 1975).

Of Arthour and of Merlin, ed. O.D. Macrae-Gibson, Early English Text Society o.s. 268, 2 vols. (London: Oxford University Press, 1973).

Of Shrifte and Penance: The Middle English Prose Translation of Le Manuel des Péchés, ed. Klaus Bitterling, Middle English Texts 29 (Heidelberg: C. Winter, 1998).

Þe *Pater Noster of Richard Ermyte*, ed. Flor Aarts, editor's proefschrift (Nijmegen: Drukkerij Gebr. Janssen, 1967).

Pearl-poet, *The Complete Works of the Pearl Poet*, trans. Casey Finch, ed. Malcolm Andrew, Ronald Waldron, and Clifford Peterson (California: University of California Press, 1993).

———, *Sir Gawain and the Green Knight, Pearl, Cleanness, Patience*, ed. J.J. Anderson (London: Dent, 1996).

Plato, *Timaeus*, trans. John Warrington (London: Dent, 1965).

Pore Caitif, ed. Sister Teresa Brady, H.D.C, unpublished PhD thesis (Fordham University, 1954).

The Prickynge of Love, ed. Harold Kane, Elizabethan and Renaissance Studies 92:10, 2 vols. (Salzburg: Institute für Anglistik und Amerikanistik, Universität Salzburg, 1983).

Pseudo-Albertus Magnus, *Women's Secrets*, trans. Helen Rodnite Lemay (Albany: State University of New York Press, 1992).

Quatrefoil of Love, ed. Israel Gollancz and Magdalene M. Weale, Early English Text Society o.s. 195 (London: Oxford University Press, 1935).

Religious Lyrics of the Fourteenth Century, ed. Carleton Brown, rev. G.V. Summers, 2nd ed. (Oxford: Clarendon Press, 1924).

The Riverside Chaucer, ed. Larry D. Benson, 3rd ed. (Boston: Houghton Mifflin Company, 1987).

Robert the Scribe, *The Bridlington Dialogue*, trans. a Religious of the Community of Saint Mary the Virgin (London: Mowbray, 1960).

Rolle, Richard, *Richard Rolle: Prose and Verse*, ed. S.J. Ogilvie-Thomson, Early English Text Society o.s. 293 (Oxford: Oxford University Press, 1988).

Saint Ambrose, *Hexameron*, trans. John Savage, Father of the Church 42 (Washington: Catholic University of America Press, 1961).

Saint Augustine of Hippo, *Basic Writings of St Augustine*, ed. Whitney J. Oates, trans. P. Holmes (New York: Random House, 1948).

———, *Christian Instruction*, trans. John J. Gavignon (Washington: Catholic University of America Press, 1947).

Saint Augustine of Hippo, *The City of God*, trans. Henry Bettenson (Harmondsworth: Penguin Books, 1972).

———, *Confessions*, trans. R.S. Pine-Coffin (Harmondsworth: Penguin Books, 1961).

———, *Expositions on the Book of Psalms*, trans. J. Tweed et al., 6 vols. (Oxford: J.H. Parker, 1847–57).

———, *Two Books on Genesis Against the Maniches*, trans. Roland J. Teske (Washington, DC: Catholic University of America Press, 1991).

Saint Thomas Aquinas, *Summa Theologiae*, 61 vols. (London: Blackfriars in conjunction with Eyre and Spottiswoode, 1964–81).

Sermons from the Worcester Chapter MS, F10, ed. Dora M. Grisdale, unpublished MA thesis, University of Leeds, 1936.

The Siege of Jerusalem, ed. E. Kölbing and Mabel Day, Early English Text Society o.s. 188 (Oxford: Oxford University Press, 1932).

Speculum Christiani, ed. Gustaf Holmstedt, Early English Text Society o.s. 182 (London: Oxford University Press, 1933 [1929]).

Speculum Sacerdotale, ed. Edward H. Weatherly, Early English Text Society o.s. 200 (London: Oxford University Press, 1936).

Stanzaic Life of Christ, ed. Frances A. Foster, Early English Text Society o.s. 166 (London: Oxford University Press, 1926).

"*Temptations*" *from Ancrene Wisse*, ed. Yoko Wada (Osaka: Institute of Oriental and Occidental Studies, Kansai University, 1994).

Theodoric of Cervia, *The Surgery of Theodoric*, trans. Eldridge Campbell and James Colton, 2 vols. (New York: Appleton-Century-Crofts, 1960).

Theophilus Presbyter, *De diversis artibus*, trans. C.R. Dodwell (London: Thomas Nelson and Sons, 1961).

Titus and Vespasian, ed. J.A. Herbert (London: J.B. Nichols, 1905).

Trevisa, John, *On the Properties of Things*, ed. M.C. Seymour, 3 vols. (Oxford: Clarendon Press, 1975–88).

———, *The English Polychronicon*, ed. Richard A. Seeger, 2 vols., unpublished PhD thesis (University of Washington, 1975).

Two Old English Apocrypha and their Manuscript Source: The Gospel of Nichodemus and the Avenging of the Saviour, ed. J.E. Cross (Cambridge: Cambridge University Press, 1997).

Vitruvius, *The Ten Books on Architecture*, trans. Morris Hicky Morgan, 2nd ed. (New York: Dover, 1960).

William of Shoreham, "The Seven Sacraments." In *The Poems of William of Shoreham*, ed. M. Konrath, Early English Text Society e.s. 86 (1902; repr. Oxford: Oxford University Press, 1975), pp. 1–78.

Yorkshire Writers, ed. C. Horstman, 2 vols. (London: Swan Sonnenschein and Co., 1896).

Secondary Sources

Amundsen, Darrel W., "Medieval Canon Law on Medical and Surgical Practice by the Clergy," *Bulletin of the History of Medicine*, 52(1978):22–45.

Anzieu, Didier, *The Skin Ego* (London: Karnac, 1989).

Arbesman, Rudolph, "The Concept of 'Christus Medicus' in St Augustine," *Traditio*, 10(1954):1–28.

Bakhtin, M.M., *The Dialogic Imagination*, ed. Michael Holquist, trans. Caryl Emerson and Michael Holquist (Austin: University of Texas Press, 1981).

Baldwin, John, "From the Ordeal to Confession: In Search of Lay Religion in Early Thirteenth-Century France." In *Handling Sin*, ed. Peter Biller and A.J. Minnis, York Studies in Medieval Theology 2 (York: York Medieval Press, 1998).

Bataille, George, *Eroticism*, trans. Mary Dalwood (London: Boyars, 1987).

Bennett, Michael, "John Audelay: Some New Evidence of his Life and Work," *The Chaucer Review*, 16:4 (1982):344–55.

Biller, Peter, "Confession in the Middle Ages: Introduction." In *Handling Sin*, ed. Peter Biller and A.J. Minnis, York Studies in Medieval Theology 2 (York: York Medieval Press, 1998).

Blanch, Robert J., and Julian N. Wasserman, *From Pearl to Gawain: Forme to Fynisment* (Gainesville, FL: University Press of Florida, 1995).

Braswell, Mary Flowers, *The Medieval Sinner* (London: Associated University Presses, 1983).

Breggner, Erik, *The Psychology of Confession*, Studies in the History of Religion 29 (Leiden: E.J. Brill, 1975).

Brzezinski, Monica, "Conscience and Covenant: The Sermon Structure of *Cleanness*," *Journal of English and Germanic Philology*, 89(1990):166–80.

Burns, E. Jane, "Speculum of the Courtly Lady," *Journal of Medieval and Early Modern Studies*, 29:2(Spring 1999):253–92.

Butler, Judith, *Bodies That Matter* (New York: Routledge, 1993).

Bynum, Caroline Walker, *Fragmentation and Redemption: Essays on Gender and the Human Body in Medieval Religion* (Zone Books: New York, 1992).

Cadden, Joan, *Meanings of Sex Difference in the Middle Ages* (New York: Cambridge University Press, 1993).

Calabrese, Michael, and Eric Eliason, "The Rhetorics of Pleasure and Sexual Intolerance in *Cleanness*," *Modern Language Quarterly*, 56(1995):247–75.

Chenu, M.-D., *Nature, Man and Society in the Twelfth Century*, ed. and trans. Etienne Gilson (Toronto: University of Toronto Press, 1997).

Cohen, Jeffrey Jerome, *Of Giants*, Medieval Cultures 17 (Minneapolis: University of Minnesota Press, 1999).

Cosman, Bard C., "All's Well That End's Well: Shakespeare's Treatment of Anal Fistula," *Diseases of the Colon and Rectum*, 41:7(1998):914–24.

Cosman, Madeleine Pelner, "Machaut's Medical Musical World." In *Machaut's World: Science and Art in the Fourteenth Century*, ed. Madeleine Pelner Cosman and Bruce Chandler (New York: New York Academy of Sciences, 1978), pp. 1–38.

Cowling, David, *Building the Text: Architecture as Metaphor in Late Medieval and Early Modern France* (Oxford: Clarendon Press, 1998).

Demaitre, Luke, "The Description and Diagnosis of Leprosy by Fourteenth-Century Physicians," *Bulletin of the History of Medicine*, 59(1985):327–44.

De Vos, Dirk, *Roger Van Der Weyden: The Complete Works* (New York: Harry N. Abrams, 1999).

Dickinson, Rev. J.C., *Origins of the Augustinian Canons and their Introduction into England* (London: Society for the Propogation of Christian Knowledge, 1950).

Dinshaw, Carolyn, *Getting Medieval: Sexualities and Communities, Pre- and Postmodern* (Durham and New York: Duke University Press, 1999).

Douglas, Mary, *Purity and Danger: An Analysis of Concepts of Pollution and Taboo* (London: Routledge and Kegan Paul, 1966).

Elliot, Dyan, "Women and Confession." In *Gendering the Master Narrative*, ed. Mary C. Erler and Maryanne Kowaleski (Ithaca and London: Cornell University Press, 2003).

Federn, Paul, *Ego Psychology and the Psychoses*, ed. Edoardo Weiss (London: Imago, 1953).

Fein, Susanna, "Good Ends in the Audelay Manuscript," *Yearbook of English Studies*, 33(2003):97–119.

Fisher, Seymour, and Sidney E. Cleveland, *Body Image and Personality* (New York: Dover Publications, 1968).

Fitzgibbons, Moira, "Disruptive Simplicity: Gaytryge's Translation of Archibishop Thoresby's *Injunctions*." In *The Vernacular Spirit*, ed. Renate Blumenfeld-Kosinski et al. (New York: Palgrave, 2002), pp. 39–57.

Fradenburg, Louise O., "Be Not Far From Me: Psychoanalysis, Medieval Studies and the Subject of Religion," *Exemplaria*, 7:1(1995):41–54.

Frankl, Paul, *The Gothic* (Princeton: Princeton University Press, 1960).

Frantzen, Allen J., "The Disclosure of Sodomy in *Cleanness*," *PMLA*, 111(1996):451–64.

Freud, Sigmund, *The Standard Edition of the Complete Psychological Works of Sigmund Freud*, ed. and trans. James Strachey et al., 24 vols. (London: Hogarth Press, 1953–74).

Gask, G.E., *Essays in the History of Medicine* (London: Butterworth and Co., 1950).

Georgianna, Linda, *The Solitary Self: Individuality in the* Ancrene Wisse (Cambridge, MA and London: Harvard University Press, 1981).

Getz, Faye, *Medicine in the English Middle Ages* (Princeton, NJ: Princeton University Press, 1998).

Gibson, Gail McMurray, "Method of Healing in Middle English," *Proceedings of the 1982 Galen Symposium*, ed. Fridolf Kudlien and Richard J. Durling (New York: E.J. Brill, 1991).

———, *The Theater of Devotion* (Chicago and London: University of Chicago Press, 1989).

Green, Richard Firth, "Marcolf the Fool and Blind John Audelay." In *Speaking Images: Essays in Honor of V.A. Kolve*, ed. Charlotte Morse and Robert F. Yeager (Asheville, NC: Pegasus Press, 2001), 559–76.

Grigsby, Bryon, *Pestilence in Medieval and Early Modern Literature* (New York and London: Routledge, 2004).

Grosz, Elizabeth, *Volatile Bodies* (Bloomington: Indiana University Press, 1994).

Hanna III, Ralph, "Contextualising *The Siege of Jerusalem*," *The Yearbook of Langland Studies*, 6(1992):109–21.

Haran, Michael, *Medieval Thought*, 2nd ed. (Toronto and Buffalo: University of Toronto Press, 1992).

Hartmann, Ernest, *Boundaries in the Mind* (New York: Basic Books, 1991).

Harvey, R.E., *The Inward Wits: Psychological Theory in the Middle Ages and Renaissance* (London: Warburg Institute, 1975).

Haubrich, William S., *Medical Meanings: A Glossary of Word Origins* (Philadelphia, PA: American College of Physicians, 1997).

Hebron, Malcolm, *The Medieval Siege* (Oxford: Clarendon Press, 1997).

Hughes, Muriel Joy, *Women Healers in Medieval Life and Literature* (Freeport: Books for Libraries Press, 1968).

Humphreys, K.W., *Books of the Austin Friars*, Corpus of British Medieval Library Catalogues (London: British Library in Association with the British Academy, 1990).

Ingledew, Francis, "Liturgy, Prophecy, and Belshazzar's Babylon: Discourse and Meaning in *Cleanness*," *Viator*, 23(1992):247–79.

Jacquart, Danielle, and Claude Thomasset, *Sexuality and Medicine in the Middle Ages*, trans. Matthew Adamson (Princeton, NJ: Princeton University Press, 1988).

Johnson, Lynn Staley, *The Voice of the Gawain-Poet* (Madison, WI: University of Wisconsin Press, 1984).

Jones, James W., *Contemporary Psychoanalysis and Religion* (New Haven:Yale University Press, 1991).

Jones, Peter Murray, "Four Middle English Translations of John Arderne." In *Latin and Vernacular*, ed. A.J. Minnis (Cambridge: D.S. Brewer, 1989), pp. 61–89.

———, "John Arderne and Surgery." In *Practical Medicine from Salerno to the Black Death*, ed. Luis García-Ballester et al. (Cambridge: Cambridge University Press, 1994), pp. 289–321.

———, "Thomas Fayreford: An English Fifteenth-Century Medical Practitioner." In *Medicine from the Black Death to the French Disease*, ed. Roger French et al. (Ashgate: Aldershot, 1998), pp. 156–83.

Karras, Ruth Mazzo, "Sharing Wine, Women, and Song: Masculine Identity Formation in the Medieval European Universities." In *Becoming Male in the Middle Ages*, ed. Jeffrey Jerome Cohen and Bonnie Wheeler (New York: Garland Publishing, 1997), pp. 187–202.

Keiser, Elizabeth B., *Courtly Desire and Medieval Homophobia* (New Haven and London: Yale University Press, 1997).

Kelly, Kathleen, "Malory's Body Chivalric," *Arthuriana*, 6:4 (1996), 52–71.

Kleinman, Arthur, *The Illness Narratives* (USA: Basic Books, 1987).

Kottek, Samuel S., *Medicine and Hygiene in the Works of Flavius Josephus* (Leiden and New York: E.J. Brill, 1994).

Kristeva, Julia, *Powers of Horror: An Essay on Abjection*, trans. Léon S. Roudiez (New York: Columbia University Press, 1982).

Kuryluk, Eve, *Veronica and her Cloth: History, Symbolism and Structure of a "True" Image* (Oxford: Oxford University Press, 1991).

Lacan, Jacques, *Écrits: A Selection*, trans. Alan Sheridan (New York: W.W. Norton, 1977).

———, "Some Reflections on the Ego," *International Journal of Psychoanalysis*, 34(1953):11–17.

Landis, Bernard, *Ego Boundaries* (New York: International Universities Press, 1970).

Lang, S.J., "John Bradmore and his Book *Philomena*," *The Social History of Medicine*, 5(1992):121–30.

Laughlin, Henry, *The Ego and its Defenses* (New York: Appleton-Century-Crofts, 1970).

Lea, Henry Charles, *The Ordeal*, ed. Edward Peters, with original documents in translation by Arthur E. Howland (Philadelphia: University of Pennsylvania Press, 1973).

Libraries of the Austin Canons, ed. T. Webber and A.G. Watson, Corpus of British Library Catalogues 6 (London: British Library in association with the British Academy, 1998).

Machan, Tim William, *Textual Criticism and Middle English Texts* (Charlottesville and London: University Press of Virginia, 1994).

McVaugh, Michael, "Therapeutic Strategies: Surgery." In *Western Medical Thought from Antiquity to the Middle Ages*, ed. Mirko D. Grmek et al. (Cambridge, MA: Harvard University Press, 1998), pp. 273–90.

Millar, Bonnie, *The Siege of Jerusalem in its Physical, Literary, and Historical Contexts* (Dublin: Four Courts Press, 2000).

Millar, T., "John Arderne, the Father of British Proctology," *Proceedings of the Royal Society of Medicine*, 47(1954):75–84.

Moe, Phyllis, "The French Source of the Alliterative *Siege of Jerusalem*," *Medium Aevum*, 39(1970):147–55.

Narin Van Court, Elisa, "*The Siege of Jerusalem* and Augustinian Historians: Writing About Jews in Fourteenth-Century England," *The Chaucer Review*, 29:3(1995):227–48.

Norri, Juhani, "Notes on the Origin and Meaning of Chemical Terms in Middle English Medical Manuscripts," *Neuphilologische Mitteilungen*, 92(1991):215–36.

Olsan, Lea, "Latin Charms in Medieval England: Verbal Healing in a Christian Oral Tradition," *Oral Tradition*, 7(1992):116–42.

Orme, Nicholas, *Medieval Children* (New Haven:Yale University Press, 2001).

Pagel-Kroll, Magda, "The Surgery of Jamerius: Report on a New Manuscript," *Bulletin of the History of Medicine*, 28(1954):471–88.

Palmer, Richard, "In Bad Odour: Smell and its Significance in Medicine from Antiquity to the Seventeenth Century." In *Medicine and the Five Senses*, ed. W.F. Bynum and Roy Porter (Cambridge: Cambridge University Press, 1993), pp. 61–68.

Paterson, Linda, "Military Surgery: Knights, Serjeants and Raimon of Avignon's Version of the *Chirurgia* of Roger of Salerno (1180–1209)." In *Ideals and Practice of Medieval Knighthood 2*, ed. Christopher Harper-Bill et al. (Suffolk: Boydell Press, 1986), pp. 117–46.

Pearsall, Derek, *Old and Middle English Poetry* (London: Routledge, 1977).

Polster, Sarah, "Ego Boundary as Process: A Systems-Contextual Approach," *Psychiatry*, 46(1983):247–58.

Porter, Roy, *The Greatest Benefit to Mankind* (London: Fontana Press, 1999).

Pouchelle, Marie-Christine, *The Body and Surgery in the Middle Ages*, trans. Rosemary Morris (New Brunswick, NJ: Rutgers University Press, 1990).

Pressman, Jack D., *Last Resort: Psychosurgery and the Limits of Medicine* (Cambridge and New York: Cambridge University Press, 1998).

The Psychological Experience of Surgery, ed. Richard S. Blacher (New York: John Wiley and Sons, 1987).

Rawcliffe, Carole, *Medicine and Society in Later Medieval England* (United Kingdom: Alan Sutton, 1995).

——, *Medicine for the Soul* (Stroud: Sutton Publishing, 1999).

——, "More Than a Bedside Manner: The Political Status of the Late Medieval Court Physician." In *St George's Chapel in the Late Middle Ages*, ed. Colin Richmond and Eileen Scarff, Historical Monographs Relating to St George's Chapel 17 (Windsor: Dean and Chapter of Windsor, 2001).

——, "On the Threshold of Eternity." In *East Anglia's History*, ed. Christopher Harper-Bill, Carole Rawcliffe, and Richard G. Wilson (Bury St Edmunds: Boydell Press, 2002), pp. 41–72.

——, *Sources for the History of Medicine in Late Medieval England* (Michigan: Medieval Institute Publications, 1995).

Raymo, Robert R., "Works of Religious and Philosophical Instruction." In *A Manual of Writings in Middle English 1050–1500*, ed. Albert E. Hartung (New Haven: The Connecticut Academy of Arts and Sciences, 1986).

Robbins, R.H., "Medical Manuscripts in Middle English," *Speculum*, 45(1970):393–415.

Root, Jerry, *"Space to Speke": The Confessional Subject in Medieval Literature* (New York: Peter Lang Publishing, 1997).

Scarry, Elaine, *The Body in Pain* (New York: Oxford University Press, 1985).

Seiler, Thomas L., "Filth and Stench as Aspects of the Iconography of Hell." In *The Iconography of Hell*, ed. Clifford Davidson and Seiler (Medieval Institute Publications: Kalamazoo, 1992).

Silvestris, Bernardus, *Commentary on the First Book of Virgil's Aeneid*, trans. Earl G. Schreiber and Thomas E. Maresca (Lincoln and London: University of Nebraska Press, 1979).

——, *Cosmographia*, trans. Winthrop Wetherbee (New York and London: Columbia University Press, 1973).

Simpson, James, *Reform and Cultural Revolution: The Oxford English Literary History Volume 2: 1350–1547* (Oxford and New York: Oxford University Press, 2002).

——, "Saving Satire after Arundel's *Constitutions*: John Audelay's 'Marcol and Solomon.' " In *Text and Controversy from Wyclif to Bale*, ed. Helen Barr and Ann Hutchison (Turnhout: Brepols, 2005), pp. 387–404.

Siraisi, Nancy, *Medieval and Renaissance Medicine: An Introduction to Knowledge and Practice* (Chicago: University of Chicago Press, 1990).

Snoeck, Andreas, *Confession and Psychoanalysis*, trans. Theodore Zuydwijk (Maryland: The Newman Press, 1964).

Spearing, A.C., *Readings in Medieval Poetry* (Cambridge: Cambridge University Press, 1987).

Stanbury, Sarah, *Seeing the "Gawain"-Poet: Description and the Act of Perception* (Philadelphia: University of Pennsylvania Press, 1991).

Stanley, Eric G., "The True Counsel of Conscience, or The Ladder of Heaven: In Defense of John Audelay's Unlyrical Lyrics." In *Expedition der Wahrheit*, ed. Stefan Horlacher and Marion Islinger (Heidelberg: Carl Winder Universitätsverlag, 1996), pp. 131–59.

Stell, Phillip, *Medical Practice in Medieval York*, Borthwick Paper 90 (York: University of York, 1996).

Taavitsainen, Irma and Päivi Pahta, eds. *Medical and Scientific Writing in Late Medieval English* (Cambridge: Cambridge University Press, 2004).

Thomas, Leo B., "Sacramental Confession and Some Clinical Concerns," *Journal of Religion and Health*, 4:4(1965):345–53.

Thornton, Martin, *English Spirituality* (London: Society for the Propagation of Christian Knowledge, 1963).

Tinkle, Theresa, "The Heart's Eye: Beatific Vision in *Purity*," *Studies in Philology*, 85(1988):451–70.

Ussery, Huling E., *Chaucer's Physician: Medicine and Literature in Fourteenth-Century England*, Tulane Studies in English 19 (New Orleans: Department of English of Tulane University, 1971).

Van Ergen, John, "Theophilus Presbyter and Rupert of Deutz," *Viator*, 2(1980):147–64.

Wallace, David, "*Cleanness* and the Terms of Terror." In *Text and Matter: New Critical Perspectives of the "Pearl"-Poet*, ed. Robert J. Blanch et al. (New York: Whitson, 1991), pp. 93–100.

Watson, Nicholas, "Censorship and Cultural Change in Late-Medieval England," *Speculum*, 70(1995):822–63.

White, Hugh, *Nature and Salvation in Piers Plowman* (Cambridge: D.S. Brewer, 1988).

White, Lynn, *Medieval Religion and Technology* (Berkeley and London: University of California Press, 1978).

Whitney, Elspeth, *Paradise Restored: The Mechanical Arts from Antiquity through to the Thirteenth Century* (Philadelphia: American Philosophical Society, 1990).

Williams, David, "Radical Therapy in *The Miller's Tale*," *The Chaucer Review*, 15(1981):227–35.

Woods, Marjorie Curry, and Rita Copeland, "Classroom and Confession." In *The Cambridge History of Medieval English Literature*, ed. David Wallace (Cambridge and New York: Cambridge University Press, 1999), pp. 376–406.

Wright, Stephen K., *The Vengeance of Our Lord: Medieval Dramatisations of the Destruction of Jerusalem* (Toronto: Pontifical Institute of Medieval Studies, 1989).

Ziegler, Joseph, *Medicine and Religion c. 1300* (Oxford: Clarendon Press, 1998).

INDEX